DISCO

D0818283

SPORTS INJURIES

After months of failure with different conventional therapies, **acupuncture** provided near miraculous results for football great Lawrence Taylor's strained left hamstring, and it works for sprains, pulled muscles, and even bone breaks!

LOWER BACK PAIN

When your hip hurts or your lower back aches, your body compensates by shifting the burden off to another area—compounding the pain! **Acupressure** helps the back muscles relax, causing the vertebrae to fall naturally into alignment—and you can administer it yourself!

MIGRAINE

Because migraines are triggered by irregular blood flow, improved circulation will lessen the pain. **Autogenic training** can stop or reduce the frequency of migraine attacks and one of the best exercises can be learned in minutes!

NEURALGIA

All over-the-counter and prescription pain relievers can have side effects. **Botanical medicines,** including horseradish, white willow bark, passion flower, hops, and valerian will give you relief that is not only effective, but safe!

PLUS

**ARTHRITIS · LOWER BACK PAIN · TMJ · CANCER PAIN
MUSCULAR AND BONE ACHES · PAIN IN THE ELDERLY**

THE DELL NATURAL MEDICINE LIBRARY
Health and Healing the Natural Way

**LOOK FOR THESE OTHER TITLES IN
THE DELL NATURAL MEDICINE LIBRARY:**

Stress, Anxiety, and Depression
Women's Health
Asthma and Allergies

THE NATURAL WAY
OF HEALING

CHRONIC
PAIN

The Natural Medicine Collective

Dr. Brian Fradet, D.C.
(Coordinating Panelist, Chiropractic)
Dr. William Bergman, M.D. *(Homeopathy)*
Brian Clement *(Nutrition)*
Elaine Retholtz, L.Ac. *(Acupuncture)*
Dr. James Lawrence Thomas, Ph.D. *(Psychology)*
Dr. Maurice H. Werness, Jr., N.D. *(Naturopathy)*

with
Theresa DiGeronimo

A DELL BOOK

PRODUCED BY THE PHILIP LIEF GROUP, INC.

Published by
Dell Publishing
a division of
Bantam Doubleday Dell Publishing Group, Inc.
1540 Broadway
New York, New York 10036

Note to the Reader:

This book is not for the purpose of self-diagnosis or self-treatment, and should be used only in conjunction with the advice of your personal doctor. Readers should consult an appropriate medical professional in all matters relating to their health.

Produced by The Philip Lief Group, Inc., 6 West 20th Street, New York, New York

ISBN: 0-440-21658-3

Printed in the United States of America

Published simultaneously in Canada

April 1995

10 9 8 7 6 5 4 3 2 1
RAD

ACKNOWLEDGMENTS

I would like to acknowledge and thank Matt DiGeronimo for his editorial assistance in all stages of researching and writing this book.

I would also like to acknowledge the help of Dominick Stampone for pulling together the bits and pieces that have now become a whole. I also thank Steve Wronko for conducting my computer searches and Eleanor Stampone for her time and effort.

The following professionals also contributed their expertise and insight:

Eli Alson, Ph.D.
Life Performance Center (biofeedback specialist)
Denville, New Jersey

Lawrence Newman, M.D.
Co-director Montefiore Headache Unit
New York, New York

Bruce Smoller, M.D.
Clinical Professor of Psychiatry
and Behavioral Sciences
George Washington University School of Medicine
Washington, D.C.

Dr. D. J. Schecter
Director, Acupuncture and Holistic Health Center
Bergenfield, New Jersey

T.D.

Contents

CHRONIC
PAIN

Introduction

Do you suffer from persistent pain? Have you seen many doctors and tried numerous medications and therapies without relief? Have you changed your lifestyle and given up things you enjoy to accommodate your pain? Are you almost out of hope? If you answer "yes" to any of these questions, natural medicine may be the key to the good health you've been looking for.

It's certainly understandable why you may be at the end of your rope. Chronic pain causes more disability than cancer and heart disease combined. It disrupts the quality of life, interferes with normal physical and social functioning, robs its victims of income and financial security, disrupts and even destroys marriages and relationships. And yet conventional medicine often does not have effective treatment.

The chronic pain patient presents physicians with a perplexing profile. In cases such as arthritis, temporomandibular joint dysfunction (TMJ), neuralgia, migraine, or cancer, the honest doctor may often say, "Your pain is caused by this specific problem, but I can't cure it or even safely stop the pain for very long." In other cases of psychogenic origin or nonspecific musculoskeletal and lower back pain, the physician often has nothing concrete to offer in way of explanation or safe treatment.

Despite the dismal prognosis, as a chronic pain patient

you have probably made the rounds of medical specialists, especially internists, orthopedists, neurologists, neurosurgeons, and psychologists/psychiatrists. Most likely, you have submitted to an endless array of costly, inexact, and time-consuming testing procedures: stool and urine analysis, blood tests, CAT (computerized axial tomography) scans, diskograms, electromyograms (EMGs), myelograms, thermograms, electroencephalograms (EEGs), venograms, MRIs (magnetic resonance imagings), and on and on. You may have tried a vast supply of expensive and addictive drugs: over-the-counter and prescription pain relievers, anti-inflammatories, antidepressants, sedatives, and tranquilizers. You may even have undergone risky surgery. Although conventional treatments from aspirin to neurosurgery do have roles to play in treating chronic pain, as you probably now know, none is without negative side effects and none is a panacea.

A key reason for your merry-go-round experience is the underlying philosophy of conventional medicine. Your physicians may have had a difficult time treating or even diagnosing your pain because typically they follow the standard approach to illness: Treat the symptoms rather than the cause. Because conventional medicine has historically slighted chronic pain as a serious disease, most research on this subject is being conducted outside the inner circle of the medical community by psychologists and neurophysiologists. These researchers are investigating how the brain controls chronic pain and how the treatment, therefore, perhaps should be focused on the brain itself rather than on the vulnerable site. Psychologists too look at pain as, at least in part, a learned function of the mind. It is known that the experience of pain is modified by emotions, memory, and learning. Psychologists are trying to tap in to the brain circuits that modify these factors and unleash their hold on pain.

Although pain research is still in its infancy, there is a large enough collection of knowledge to give you sound reasons to rethink your treatment approach. The failure of drugs and surgery in treating most forms of chronic pain does not signal the demise of hope—it sounds a call to look in new directions. Alternative therapies use what we know about the relationship between the brain and pain and the mental power we each possess to control this connection. It is these alternatives that we discuss in this book. Here you'll learn that you've not reached the end; you've just begun a new adventure. You'll find that the quality-of-life factor is a paramount concern in natural treatment therapies—no more ghastly side effects, no more social isolation, no more passive acceptance of invasive treatment. Through the pages of this book you'll learn how to help put yourself in charge of your own pain.

We realize that you may come to this information a bit skeptical, and with good reason. You have, either personally or through discussion, learned of the disappointing results in conventional chronic pain treatments. It's no wonder you may now think "What's the use? Nothing will work." An interesting study comparing the beliefs of patients visiting a general practitioner and a homeopath found that most patients turned to natural medicine only after being frustrated with conventional medicine. Unfortunately, this long-term experience with frustration can keep you from using alternative remedies confidently and conscientiously, thus sabotaging your quest for a pain-free existence.

Through the pages of this book, we hope to give you back your confidence and encourage you to explore the use of alternative remedies conscientiously. We hope to give you a positive attitude toward natural medicine that's based on knowledge; this will allow you to "prove" to yourself the worth of this natural approach to chronic pain.

The first chapter, "The World of Chronic Pain," discusses the physiological and psychological aspects of pain. This chapter differentiates between acute pain (the specialty of conventional medicine) and chronic pain (the bane of modern medicine). It then explains how pain works: what happens in the body when you feel pain, what makes it stop, and why it sometimes continues. You'll learn why the appropriate and effective acute pain therapies are often dismal failures in the treatment of chronic pain. Chapter 1 also explores the relationship between the mind and the body. You will see how the depression caused by chronic pain creates more pain and begins a cycle that can keep you incapacitated and isolated. And finally, this chapter encourages you to let natural remedies break the cycle. You are challenged to proceed with an open mind and a determined will to take charge of your own body, health, and pain.

Chapter 2, "What Is Natural Medicine?," introduces you to the world of alternative remedies. You will learn about the differences between conventional and natural medicine. You will explore the history of natural healing. The training and licensing of naturopathic doctors is explained. And finally you'll learn how to locate a physician of natural medicine. With this informative background, you'll be better able to appreciate and understand the specific natural therapies explained in Chapter 3.

In part, Chapter 3 is an overview of the most common forms of natural medicine that anyone investigating this approach to healing should know of. These include: acupuncture and acupressure, homeopathy, hydrotherapy, herbalism, nutrition, chiropractic manipulation, massage, reflexology, exercise, psychotherapy, relaxation techniques, hypnosis, and transcutaneous electrical nerve stimulation (TENS). Then, where appropriate within this general overview, certain therapies are discussed in detail to give a complete picture of how that remedy can be used effectively in the treatment of pain. As the therapies are later applied to specific pain syndromes, you will be asked to refer back to this chapter.

Chapters 4 through 12 look at very specific kinds of pain. Although the information regarding the use of natural medicine applies to all kinds of pain, we felt it would be of value to you to separate out the most common and debilitating sources of chronic pain. These include: arthritis, lower back pain, migraine headaches, TMJ, neurogenic pain, cancer pain, generalized musculoskeletal pain, psychogenic pain, and pain in the elderly. In these chapters you'll learn what researchers know about the cause of your pain, why it's so resistant to conventional cures, and what the future may hold for its treatment. Then the natural remedies discussed in Chapter 3 that have tested as effective for each type of pain are discussed.

Finally, be sure to read Chapter 13 on the growing popularity and use of pain clinics. As chronic pain gains a place in the medical community as a serious condition warranting full medical attention, these clinics are popping up all over the country. This chapter fills you in on their use and abuse.

As you can see, this book is full of informative and useful material. But knowing the facts is not enough to ease your pain. We have put this book together to help you *do* something about the pain that is keeping you from living the productive and fulfilling life you deserve. Our goal in advocating these alternative therapies is to help you find a way to reduce your pain and suffering with minimal or no side effects. But most important, we want to give you the means by which you can become an active participant in your own health care.

One important note to keep in mind: The information in this book is not intended to replace your traditional medical care. It should be used only in conjunction with the advice of your physician. You should always consult your doctor before undertaking any treatment or making any medical-related decisions.

As you read through each chapter, try to remember that you don't want to focus so intently on your pain that it becomes your primary thought. You want to achieve just the opposite: Let natural medicine help your body and mind to give up its obsession with pain, and move on to experiencing the many joys of life.

CHAPTER ONE

The World of Chronic Pain

Pain—everyone experiences it, yet no one is able to describe it precisely. No two people experience it in exactly the same way, and science has yet to find a way to measure it accurately. Although ever-changing, mysterious, and indescribable, pain does have a function: It lets us know when something is wrong and it insists that the problem be rectified immediately. Pain that screams and demands attention is known as *acute* pain. Although even the thought of this piercing discomfort alone is enough to make us cringe, it is actually beneficial to our body's health. In fact, acute pain is not a problem at all, just the identifier of one. Take the case of the person with no feeling in her hand; when she places that hand on a hot stove, she won't remove it from the scorching sting instantly because she feels no pain. Although in theory the idea of feeling no pain sounds desirable, let us not be envious—the hand will have suffered severe, perhaps irreparable, damage. As smoke detectors are used to sense fire in its infancy, so too acute pain is only the detector, not the fire.

In other cases, however, pain is like a wayward fire siren —a relentless and unforgiving signal of distress, refusing to silence even when the fire is out. When a specific pain continues to be unresponsive to treatment for more than six months, it's then classified as *chronic* pain. Chronic pain, as approximately 65 million Americans know, is all-consuming, affecting much more than just physical health. Its insidious tentacles can reach out to entwine in its grasp one's emotional and mental health, along with even financial and marital well-being.

Despite its age-old grip on the quality of a sufferer's life, only recently has chronic pain been recognized by the conventional medical community as a severe problem in and of itself. Still, in many thousands of cases, its treatment remains a conundrum for medical experts. Standard treatments for the ceaseless pain of arthritis, neuralgia, cancer, and old age, for example, are too often temporary, ineffectual, or even dangerous.

Many medical professionals fail to recognize that chronic pain problems are complex in nature and generally involve much more than subjective experience of pain. The patient's overall pain experience is augmented by additional pain-related symptoms. Associated symptoms and problems are at least as important as the perceived pain. This is typically referred to as chronic pain syndrome. To determine if you may be experiencing this syndrome, ask yourself the following questions.

1. Do you have persistent pain despite multiple medical interventions?
2. Do you exhibit observable pain behaviors such as moaning, limping, complaining, and the like?
3. Do you have a functional impairment?
4. Do you have an overreliance on pain-relief devices, medications, or activities?
5. Do you suffer emotional distress related to the pain?
6. Do you notice a disruption in your interpersonal relationships?

If you find yourself answering "yes" to these questions, then you need to know that to treat chronic pain conditions effectively, all of these symptoms, not just the symptom of pain, must be addressed.

This failure of modern medicine is perplexing to chronic pain sufferers. We have grown up in a society that we tend to think has an instant medical cure for everything. TV commercials assure us, "Have a headache? Take a pill." "Have a cold or the flu? Take this for quick symptomatic relief." And true to their claims, many medications do "cure" our ills time and time again. But chronic pain is different. Suddenly there is no promise of relief, no quick cures, and then, seemingly, no hope.

For centuries natural remedies that focus on diet, exercise, state of mind, and natural meridians of the body have been proven effective in treating chronic pain. Now as we approach the twenty-first century, these therapies are getting a well-deserved second look. By combining what we have learned about pain through modern technological advances with what has been known throughout time by natural healers, we now can substantiate and validate remedies that in the American medical community have lived under the shadow of quackery. And so the chronic pain patient now has a new vision of hope.

Your venture into natural medicine will be most beneficial and productive if you understand why you hurt and how natural remedies ease the pain. Let's take a look at what causes pain, why we feel it, and how our body tries to defend against it.

THE PHYSIOLOGY OF PAIN

When you stub your toe, the pain you feel is not really coming from your toe. Pain is a function of the central nervous system that is processed through the brain—it is therefore in the brain that you actually feel the pain caused by your injury. Many of the pain-control techniques presented later in this book require that you understand this, so it certainly is worth repeating. Say it out loud and remember: The sensation of pain is a function of the brain.

A persuasive example of this fact is offered by Indian fakirs. These "wonder workers," as they are sometimes called, lie on beds of nails and walk across hot coals without experiencing the pain we would expect these actions to cause. It is not that there is anything exceptional about the strength of their backs or feet; they can withstand these rituals because they have mastered the skill of *mental* pain control. An overview of the biological process of pain will help explain why some natural remedies succeed where conventional medicine fails.

You can think of the brain and nervous system as a complex communications network. The messenger units of this network are biochemical substances called neurotransmitters; they carry the body's internal communications. The migration of the neurotransmitters to the brain is initiated by small nerve cells, called nociceptors, that are located all over the body. When the nociceptors sense physical danger, they send two signals to the brain. One piece of information is sent directly and quickly to the brain to identify the location of the danger and determine what action is needed to rectify the situation.

The second message transmits a neurotransmitter, known as substance P, on a longer and less direct path up the spine to the brain cell neurons. The neurons identify substance P with their antennalike structures, called dendrites, and connect with the neurotransmitter in a lock-and-key fashion. The neuron then fires a biochemical mixture that contains more substance P, which proceeds to find more receptive neurons; the result is a chain reaction that causes the sensation of pain.

This process is what makes pain a subjective experience. When we're hurt, the brain instantly judges whether the injury signals a threat to our well-being. Only afterward does it try to determine exactly what happened and where the injury exists. (This sequence of subjective experience followed by objective naming happens also with our sense of smell and taste.)

You may have witnessed these two pain signals at work in your own body. Have you ever cut yourself badly with a knife, quickly dropped the knife in horror, and then looked at a gaping wound in your hand, realizing that you haven't yet felt any pain? This happens because the nociceptor shot the danger message to the brain to drop the knife and stop the damage to the hand—this was the more urgent message. The body's first priority is self-preservation; in a case like this, your body first uses its energy to remove the danger. Then substance P arrives a few seconds later and the sensation of pain soon follows.

The arrival of substance P is slightly delayed because it must first pass through a "gate" at the bottom of the spinal cord. This gate, discovered by the revolutionary studies of Canadian scientists Drs. Patrick Wall and Ronald Melzack, must open to allow substance P to enter. *In cases of acute pain,* the gate opens to allow substance P access to the brain; then as the body begins to heal, it reduces the amount allowed to enter. This too is part of the body's ability to make sure we listen to our pain. The pain of a broken leg, for example, ensures that the leg will be given time to heal before it is required to hold the weight of the body again. As the bone heals, the pain will lessen bit by bit, allowing the injured person to put increasingly more and more weight on the leg.

When the pain signal is sounded for the release of substance P, another type of neurotransmitter also is released to play the role of substance P's nemesis—endorphins, meaning "morphine within." These newly discovered natural painkillers are produced by the brain and oppose the effects of substance P. An interesting characteristic of these natural painkillers is that they too sit at the base of the spinal cord waiting for a signal to pass through the gate, and they also fit brain cell neurons with the same lock-and-key mechanism as does substance P.

By attaching to neurons, endorphins interrupt the pain-causing chain reaction of substance P because they reduce the number of neurons substance P can hook up to. When endorphins gain a strong hold on the neurons, pain dissipates.

Morphine works in a very similar manner, but endorphins are a more desirable source of pain control for a number of reasons:

- They are ten times more effective than morphine.
- They never lose their potency as do analgesic drugs.
- They are safer because the body produces them naturally and therefore there is no risk of addiction.

Research has discovered what signals the gate mechanism response to substance P and endorphins. Under the normal circumstances brought on by acute pain, endorphins flood the gate and form a barricade against substance P. Like two armies of equal strength and numbers, neither moves the other one back. However, when the nociceptors release more substance P, the battle becomes lopsided and substance P continues to pass up the spinal cord, causing the sensation of pain until the body feels it is out of danger. When the danger to the body is removed or an injury heals, the numbers of endorphins and substance P return to normal and the gate closes until the next time a physical injury occurs.

In the case of chronic pain, the process is the same with one exception. The body's physical response to pain still involves the battle between substance P and endorphins, but for a variety of reasons (some of which are still unclear), the gate doesn't close when the battle is over. Pain signals are allowed continuous access to the brain. Dr. Bruce Pomeranz, a neurophysiologist at the University of Toronto, feels that chronic pain may involve a learning process in the nervous system. He believes that if you have repeated pain inputs coming into the nervous system, in some way they become engraved or carved in stone, so the pain persists long after the lesion is gone. The pain circuits are firing by themselves—they no longer need inputs from the diseased organ. Naturally, this "cause" of pain will resist conventional medical treatment at the affected site.

Whatever the exact cause of chronic pain, this alteration of the natural course of events makes diagnosing and treating the condition difficult.

THE FAILURE OF
CONVENTIONAL MEDICINE

Many American medical doctors in certain specialty areas are the best in the world. Medical research and modern technology offer today's patient modes of prevention, miraculous cures, and reasons for hope in the treatment of diseases and ailments that, in some cases, even ten years ago would have been fatal. In the realm of chronic pain, however, conventional American medicine has failed millions of sufferers. With sincere intent and state-of-the-art expertise, medical experts try relentlessly to silence the siren of ceaseless pain, but unfortunately the tools available to them do not offer long-term relief for most pain sufferers.

Only two common modes of pain treatment are available to chronic pain sufferers through conventional medical channels: drugs and surgery.

Drug Therapy

The pharmacological store of pain-relief drugs is immense. There are drugs to ease pain, inflammation, depression, and anxiety. There are over-the-counter drugs, prescription nonnarcotic drugs, and narcotic drugs. Unfortunately, none has yet been found that can offer long-term relief without dangerous side effects.

Over-the-Counter Drugs

The most commonly used nonprescription drug for pain relief is aspirin. Aspirin (also known as a salicylate) is a relatively safe drug and is most effective in the treatment of various kinds of musculoskeletal and inflammatory pain such as rheumatic and arthritic disorders and tension headaches. However, if taken in high doses for long periods of time, aspirin can be quite harmful.

Aspirin abuse can cause gastric irritation, which may lead to ulceration and hemorrhage. It also can affect the liver, resulting in defects of the blood-clotting mechanism and metabolic functions, with loss of such important substances as amino acids through the kidneys. Painless bleeding through the stools is seen occasionally even with low aspirin dosages and can result in iron-deficiency anemia. The most frightening symptoms of aspirin abuse are those affecting the nervous system: dizziness, ringing in the ears, drowsiness, visual disturbances, and deafness. Often these side effects are not associated with aspirin intake and prompt the patient to seek further medical help and medications for these new "illnesses."

Recognizing the drawbacks of aspirin for pain relief, the pharmaceutical industry turned to production of over-the-counter "aspirin-free" pain relievers. The most commonly used of these are acetaminophen and ibuprofen. Acetaminophen is the active ingredient found in the popular product Tylenol. Unfortunately, acetaminophen does not have the anti-inflammatory action of aspirin that so successfully treats the inflamed joints of acute arthritis and other inflammatory distress syndromes. In addition, prolonged use of this drug also can be quite harmful to the liver.

Ibuprofen is the active ingredient in the pain relievers Advil, Nuprin, Excedrin IB, and Motrin. All contain 200 milligrams of ibuprofen. Filler ingredients, which may differ, do not alter the effectiveness of the pain-relieving drug. Because all of these over-the-counter drugs contain the same active ingredient, you can expect the same negative side effects. This drug may be irritating to the stomach and intestines, and it also may produce blurred or diminished vision. Although quite effective for short-term relief, the gastrointestinal effects make ibuprofen a poor choice for chronic pain relief.

All analgesics—aspirin, nonaspirin, prescription, and nonprescription—can cause "rebound" pain. Rebound pain is that pain actually caused by the frequent use of analgesics. When analgesics are taken too often, the body may adapt to having pain relievers in the system at all times. When the pain relief begins to wear off, the awareness of pain becomes greater. When this happens, the patient either will strengthen the rebound effect by taking more analgesics or will look to stronger, narcotic-based drugs for relief.

Narcotics

Narcotics are useful drugs when used to treat acute pain. However, under no circumstances should any narcotic be prescribed without a definite plan for its discontinuation. For the chronic pain patient, then, this category of drug should be automatically eliminated from consideration; by its very definition, "chronic" means without end. All narcotics have the potential for causing tolerance, addiction, and withdrawal; not only are they inappropriate for long-term use, but they are dangerous when given over a period of time.

Opiates are sometimes prescribed to relieve chronic pain despite the fact that long-term use can cause serious complications, addiction, and untold misery for the patient. Many drugs are included in this category of opiates, including natural derivatives such as morphine and codeine, chemical derivatives of morphine and codeine such as heroin, and synthetic opiates such as pethidine (Demerol) and methadone.

Tolerance to opiates grows rapidly; in just a few days after initial use, a larger dosage may be needed to produce the same effect. As tolerance builds, patients must take the drug almost constantly to avoid unpleasant withdrawal symptoms.

As the dosage is increased, the negative side effects of opiates also are increased. Long-term use of these narcotics often results in constipation, urinary retention, constriction of the lung's air passages, and low blood pressure.

Barbiturates

Barbiturates have no direct pain-relief action. However, frequently they are prescribed as sleeping aids for patients whose pain keeps them awake at night. These too rapidly produce tolerance and are highly addictive. Many times barbiturates are combined with pain-relief medication such as aspirin to serve dual duty—pain reduction and sedation. This combination, however, is dangerous because a person in pain may take more and more pills to gain physical relief, not realizing that the barbiturate abuse will wreak havoc with the sleep cycle, making it more difficult to sleep, and also cause impairment of judgment and coordination. Additionally, a side effect of habitual barbiturate use is depression, which (as discussed in greater detail later) can actually increase and prolong pain.

Tranquilizers

Tranquilizers can help a chronic pain patient rest without narcotics. They also can provide some indirect pain relief by reducing muscle tension, which can aggravate pain. Commonly prescribed tranquilizers are the benzodiazepines, which include diazepam (Valium) and chlordiazepoxide (Librium). When properly used for short-term, acute cases, these drugs are effective and safe. However, they generally cause more problems than they remedy in the chronic pain patient.

Tranquilizers also eventually produce tolerance and addiction. Like barbiturates, in large doses they can cause impairment of judgment and coordination. They also can cause depression and a sense of helplessness that keeps the pain patient from taking control of the pain and being actively involved in finding a way to live comfortably. Too often tranquilizers are used without the accompanying psychotherapy that would teach the patient how to relax and find a sense of well-being without the use of drugs.

Nerve blocks are another way of delivering drug therapy. Injections into what are called "trigger points" offer relief for many who suffer the chronic pain of specific conditions, such as lumbar muscle strain or myofascial syndrome. An injection of a local anesthetic into a specific body point blocks pain messengers from the injured area from reaching the brain. If you have ever received an injection of Novocain during dental work, you have experienced a trigger-point injection and know how effective it can be in stopping the sensation of pain.

Although effective, this pharmacological approach to pain relief also has its problems. The relief lasts only as long as or slightly longer than the effects of the anesthesia. If you're an outpatient, this can mean returning to your physician for an injection every day. Also, trigger-point injections treat only the symptom of pain, not the cause, so the pain always will return. Moreover, because a trigger-point injection can aggravate the condition, often the pain returns with more intensity than before. And finally, the body can develop a tolerance for the anesthesia, requiring more frequent injections with reduced effect.

Surgery

Surgery of any kind is always risky. There is the ever-present danger of excessive bleeding, infection, and damage to other organs. Anesthesia carries with it risks of heart, lung, and other complications that are potentially fatal. Still, for the treatment of many diseases and ailments, surgery is sometimes absolutely necessary. For the chronic pain patient, however, surgery is almost never necessary or desirable.

Surgeons are schooled to treat with a knife; chronic pain patients continually find that if they go to a surgeon for advice, they come home with stitches.

There are two kinds of pain surgery: surgery directed at

the cause of the pain, and surgery directed at the nerves that carry the pain to the brain. The first type includes surgery for specific problems, such as a herniated disk or a tumor. Because there is a clearly definable reason for treatment with surgery, this approach to pain is commonly prescribed and generally safe and effective.

Perhaps the most commonly performed and least successful type of surgery for chronic pain is the second kind —neurosurgery. Four kinds of neurosurgery are practiced commonly today:

1. Dorsal Rizotomy: This is a neurosurgical procedure in which the surgeon cuts the roots of the nerves connecting the spinal cord with a specific part of the anatomy.

2. Cordotomy: In this procedure, the neurosurgeon inserts an electric needle into the spinal cord and congeals the nerve tract that carries fibers from the affected area through the spine to the brain.

3. Tractotomy: Particularly suited to shoulder and neck pain, in this procedure the neurosurgeon interrupts the nerve fibers in the area of the brain stem, well above the spinal cord.

4. Electrostimulation: In an attempt to make the nerves resistant to pain, in this procedure the neurosurgeon inserts an electric needle into the spinal cord and stimulates the nerve fibers.

Although the short-term results of neurosurgery often offer dramatic relief from pain, the long-term results are disheartening. Nerve-severing surgery may eliminate not only pain, but other sensations as well. The patient may lose feeling for warmth, coolness, or taste, for example. Neurosurgery for pain also is known to cause new problems. After the nerve is cut, many patients report burning pains in the part of the body served by the cut nerve. Surgeons can't predict or avoid these outcomes in certain patients.

And finally, and most discouraging, it's not at all uncommon for the original pain to return several months after the surgery. How the pain finds a new way to get through to the brain, or what exact route it takes after the messenger nerve is cut, it unknown at this time, but it certainly does happen, making neurosurgery a very risky course of treatment for the chronic pain patient. Long-term follow-up studies are sufficiently discouraging to indicate that nerve-altering surgery should not be used in the management of chronic pain.

Another invasive approach to the treatment of chronic pain is electrode implants. These electrodes can be surgically placed just behind the spinal cord to cause electrically stimulated interference with the passage of substance P through the gate mechanism. Or they can be implanted in certain areas of the brain itself to electrically stimulate an increased endorphin production. The electrode is connected to leads implanted under the skin at a convenient site; the lead is connected to a portable device outside the body that allows the patient to activate and control the electrical stimulation. Dramatic, positive results have been reported by chronic pain patients who suddenly find they can control their own pain with just a turn of the voltage dial.

Electrical stimulation has proven to be very effective initially for about two out of three patients. But in addition to the risks involved in any type of surgery, extended use of this expensive option has proven disappointing in long-term studies. It seems that as the brain becomes accustomed to the electrical stimulations, larger and larger doses are required to achieve the desired pain relief. However, the apparatus is designed to discharge only a certain amount of voltage. Once the brain craves voltage that exceeds this maximum amount, the electrodes are ineffectual and the patient is back to square one. This effect is analogous to the brain's reaction to drugs such as morphine; eventually the morphine's effect will be minimal and the patient is left in pain with an addiction.

Drugs and surgery—the two cornerstones of conventional medicine's approach to pain—have failed the chronic pain patient too often. This failure is key to the appearance of psychological problems that further aggravate pain.

THE PSYCHOLOGICAL INJURY OF CHRONIC PAIN

In many cases the physical symptom of pain is only one contributing factor to the creation of the abysmal and turbulent cycle chronic pain sufferers find themselves caught in. Although this cycle begins and ends with physical suffering, it is powered by psychological aspects of chronic pain. The most detrimental of these is depression. Although the exact relationship between depression and chronic pain remains ambiguous, experts have no doubt that depression increases the perception of pain and decreases one's tolerance for pain.

It's understandable why the chronic pain sufferer is prone to depression. An individual who suffers from chronic pain hopes desperately for an accurate diagnosis with an effective treatment. Oftentimes the patient has seen several doctors, consumed a variety of medications, undergone surgery, and spent much time and money—all to no avail. Clearly this is an understandable cause of depression.

In addition, chronic pain sufferers fall into depression

because they tend to regress from normal, everyday activities. They often withdraw from both physical and social functions, giving themselves more reason to feel alone and depressed. They may give pain the upper hand, relinquish all life's responsibilities, and become completely dependent on others for their survival.

Often the chronic pain patient's treatment aggravates an already depressed psychological state. Depression is a well-known side effect of strict bed rest, surgery, and many commonly prescribed pain medications.

Under these circumstances, it's no wonder that chronic pain is so often wed to depression. Unfortunately, this marriage of pain and depression can begin a far-reaching psychosomatic chain reaction. When pain is not alleviated promptly and the sufferer becomes disturbed emotionally, the body's response to this disturbance may show itself in physiological symptoms such as nausea, gastrointestinal disease, or stress reactions such as headaches, heart palpitations, anxiety attacks, or dizziness. The occurrence of suffering, distinct from the pain itself, compounds the feeling of helplessness. In the face of a seemingly endless course of deteriorating health, many find themselves victims of depression, personality changes, and even suicidal fantasies.

The physical response to psychological problems is often the result of depression's effect on the immune system. University of Iowa psychiatrist Dr. Ziad Kronfel has proven that the immune systems of depressed people are substantially less responsive than those of normal individuals or patients having other mental diseases. Other follow-up studies have supported this finding. So here we see how the cycle is set into motion. The chronic pain causes depression. Depression weakens the immune system, causing physical problems unrelated to the original pain. As the state of health deteriorates further, the depression worsens, aggravating the pain condition.

Consider how you mentally manage your pain. Do you think about your pain? Concentrate on its intensity? Listen to your body for signals of coming pain? Well, if you do, consider this analogy that demonstrates how your mental focus may be keeping you locked in the cycle of pain.

Imagine there is a creaking gate outside your window. If you are busy working around the house, the creaking of the gate will go unnoticed—never registering in your conscious mind. Now imagine you are not busy. You are lying in bed and all is silent, except for the creaking gate. The gate will soon catch your attention and dominate your every thought. You'll listen for it, anticipate it, picture it, focus on it, until eventually you feel you can't stand it anymore.

In the same way, you may tend to listen to the creaks of your body more intensely as depression increases and activity decreases. It is well known that depression increases pain perception and decreases pain tolerance. This gives you one more reason to feel depressed and keep the cycle in motion.

This worst-case scenario shows how chronic pain patients sometimes surrender to a life of misery and suffering without trying to help themselves out of it—thus creating a self-fulfilling prophesy. But this doesn't have to be the case with you. You *can* explore ways to control your own pain and live the kind of life you long for.

BREAKING THE CYCLE
WITH NATURAL MEDICINE

Natural medicine will help you put together a treatment plan that takes into account the role of the body and the mind in pain control. Without invasive therapies, addictive drugs, or costly medical tests and procedures, the remedies presented in this book will help you take charge of your pain and accept responsibility for managing it.

Chapter Two

What Is
Natural Medicine?

Acid rain . . . the disappearing ozone layer . . . smog . . . radiation . . . contaminated well water . . . It has become evident, from media reports as well as from personal experiences, that our increasing knowledge and technology can both help to advance society as well as wreak havoc on our lives. In a similar way, as the science of medicine has become more technical and has made great strides in treating many illnesses, it also has become more and more manipulative of and invasive to the human body. Unnecessary surgeries, excessive medication, life-support mechanisms . . . all of these alter the natural processes of health and illness, life and death. One cannot deny the value of surgery and medication in treating certain ailments and diseases, but it seems that we often lose sight of the body's power and ability, with the proper care and nurturing, to heal itself.

This notion of healing oneself is at the root of natural medicine philosophy. As more people witness the harmful effects of technology and the overuse of conventional modern medicine, they are turning to alternatives that are less invasive and disruptive of the body's natural processes. The "health-consciousness craze" of the 1990s is all around us. People are striving to eat the right foods and maintain their proper weight; more people have made exercise a regular part of their daily routine; and some have discovered the benefits of relaxation and meditation, two elements that are particularly vital in our fast-paced, hectic lives.

You might grant that diet, exercise, and stress reduction are all well and good, yet doubt that they are a sufficient means of curing specific illnesses. How can riding the Lifecycle for twenty minutes three times a week possibly help chronic acid indigestion? The missing link is the mind: Proper care of your body helps create a healthy mind, and a balanced mind leads to a healthy body. They are interrelated; some believe they are one and the same. As a society, we are skeptical—we like to have things proven through testing and experimentation, and we like to see the facts. The brain and neurological system can be viewed as the physical embodiment of the mind, and this is true to the extent that scientists and doctors can measure and test these vital organs. The mind, however, is more than a mass of nerves, hormones, and electrical impulses. It represents an invisible, intangible, yet extremely powerful energy that, unfortunately, we often are too quick to dismiss.

Throughout history the mind has been viewed as something that must be mastered and controlled, otherwise one might "lose one's mind" or "go out of one's mind." An inability to control one's mind signified personal weakness to many people. It is useful, however, to think of the mind not as something to be controlled lest one go mad, but as energy to be harnessed and used to restore and maintain overall health. Indeed, this is the underlying philosophy of the practice of natural medicine.

Vis medicatrix naturae—the healing power of nature— this is the premise of natural medicine, which involves the use of an array of noninvasive natural therapies to help restore balance to the body and thus help the system to heal itself. These therapies, which will be discussed individually in Chapter 3, include Oriental medicine, homeopathy, hydrotherapy, botanical medicine, physical medicine, psychotherapy, biofeedback, and nutrition. Natural medicine discourages the use of treatments that weaken the body's innate ability to heal itself, and although a person sometimes requires more than natural remedies, the natural medicine practitioner will always try to use the least invasive treatment possible.

Natural medicine functions from a holistic point of view; that is, your whole being is treated, rather than simply the part of your body that is sick. Natural medicine practitioners will take into consideration not only your obvious and immediate symptoms but lifestyle, psychological factors, and other physical imbalances that may be present. They believe that illness affects the whole person—physically, emotionally, and mentally—and that imbalances within and among these three spheres will cause a person to exhibit symptoms of sickness. Natural medicine requires you to become involved in your own healing and to claim responsibility for your own health. Doctors have long been considered teachers of a certain kind, and natural medicine practitioners continue the tradition of educating their patients to become more aware of their own bodies, emotions, and minds and to help the self-healing process along.

Natural medicine strives for a balance between mind and body. If appropriate and necessary, various therapies can be used concurrently, or they can be used to supplement standard medical treatment if the case warrants it. The fact is that no one remedy or therapy—whether it is conventional or alternative—can work for everyone all of the time. The key is to explore your options and use the treatment that is most successful in treating your overall health and well-being.

Natural therapies are gaining popularity as people increasingly realize that conventional medicine cannot always offer all the answers or cures. According to a study published in the *New England Journal of Medicine* in January 1993, approximately one-third of all Americans used alternative medicine therapies in 1990, including relaxation techniques, massage, macrobiotic diets, spiritual healing, self-help groups, biofeedback, acupuncture, hypnosis, chiropractic, herbal medicine, and homeopathy. Patients spent $10.3 billion on alternative health care in 1990, and 90 percent of the treatments were sought by patients without the advice or suggestion of their regular physician.

The mainstream health-care industry, likewise, is changing to keep up with the growing demand for alternative medicine. The National Institutes of Health, at the urging of Congress, established an Office for the Study of Unconventional Medicine Practices and an Office of Alternative Medicine in 1992. Some conventional physicians have incorporated natural medicine philosophy and techniques into their own practices. Insurance companies such as the American Western Life Insurance Company of California, the Mutual of Omaha Insurance Company, Blue Cross of Washington and Alaska, and the New Jersey–based Prudential have extended coverage to include natural therapies. Clearly, natural medicine is becoming more popular as patients seek alternative treatments to those offered in Western medicine.

DIFFERENCES BETWEEN CONVENTIONAL AND ALTERNATIVE MEDICINE

Standard, conventional, or orthodox medicine, also called *allopathy,* defines health as the absence of disease. This definition is based on a negative. In contrast, holistic medicine concurs with the definition of health used by the

World Health Organization (WHO), which posits that it is a state of complete physical, mental, and social well-being.

The allopathic and holistic definitions of health differ greatly in regard to the diagnosis and treatment of illness. People who use conventional medicine usually do not seek treatment until they become ill; there is little emphasis on preventive treatment. Holistic medicine, in contrast, focuses on preventing illness and maintaining health. The best illustration of this approach is the fact that ancient Chinese doctors were paid only when their patients were healthy, not if they became ill.

Natural medicine, which follows a holistic approach, views illness and disease as an imbalance of the mind and body that is expressed on the physical, emotional, and mental levels of a person. Although allopathy does recognize that many physical symptoms have mental components (for example, emotional stress might promote an ulcer or chronic headaches), its approach is generally to suppress the symptoms, both physical and psychological. Natural medicine assesses the symptoms as a sign or reflection of a deeper instability within the person, and it tries to restore the physical and mental harmony that will then alleviate the symptoms.

Except for cases of severe physical trauma, most illness derives from a level of susceptibility that varies in different people. For instance, some people seem to catch every cold and flu virus that goes around, while others can go for years without so much as a sniffle or a cough. The level of susceptibility reflects the deepest state of one's being. Bacteria and germs, as well as carcinogens, allergens, and other toxins, are agents of illness waiting to prey on a susceptible host. These stimuli alone do not cause illness, but rather induce specific symptoms in susceptible persons. Certain bacteria are known to be associated with certain diseases, and there are bacteria living within our bodies all of the time. Hence, if bacteria were the cause of illness, we would probably be sick all of the time. Instead, illness occurs when an imbalance in the body allows the bacteria to reproduce uncontrollably. Natural medicine usually views this uncontrolled growth as a manifestation of disease, not a cause of it. Natural medicine practitioners believe that preventive medicine, or therapies designed to maintain and enhance health, can reduce people's susceptibility and therefore the frequency with which they become ill.

Because of the fundamental differences in the way that allopathic and alternative physicians define and view health and illness, they also assess and treat their patients in very different ways. Alternative practitioners believe that people can use the power and positive energy of their minds to defend themselves against disease. Symptoms, therefore, are not caused by illness, but reflect the body's best attempt to heal itself. Since allopathic doctors believe that symptoms are caused by disease, they also believe that alleviating the symptoms will foster cure. In contrast, the natural medicine practitioner will claim that suppressing symptoms fails to address the underlying cause of illness and, in fact, can drive the illness deeper into the body, causing more profound symptoms to develop.

For example, if a child has a fever, an allopathic doctor might prescribe acetaminophen. Although this can help to bring the fever down, it is not curing the illness, which must run its course. An alternative practitioner, on the other hand, would consider the fever to be an indication that the body is fighting the illness. A high temperature makes the body unsuitable for bacteria to grow, and so it is the body's natural defense against the infection. Of course, an excessively high fever can be dangerous and should be treated so as to reduce it.

The difference between allopathic and natural treatments also can be seen in relation to the common cold. An allopathic doctor might suggest using an antihistamine to dry up a runny nose. However, natural medicine believes that the flow of mucus, and indeed all bodily secretions, is significant to the healing process, as it rids the body of toxic substances. If you are the kind of person who likes the quick remedy—that magic syrup or pill—and does not want to endure the discomforts of illness in the recovery process, you will have to assess whether natural medicine is appropriate for you. All of the alternative therapies discussed in this book require that your mind be open to their philosophies and that you become an active participant in your own recovery and health promotion.

In allopathy, diagnostic testing is vital in order for the doctor to name and categorize the disease and to treat it. Often these tests are done routinely, sometimes for the purpose of protecting the doctor rather than actually to help the patient. Some diagnostic tests, such as excessive X rays, or the use of powerful drugs can even cause sickness, referred to as iatrogenic illness, meaning "doctor-caused."

Although modern holistic doctors might use some standard diagnostic tests, they are more concerned with the individual's life circumstances. When you visit an alternative practitioner for the first time, he or she will consult at length with you, or "take the case," as it is called. During this initial visit, which can last more than an hour, the doctor will interview you, making notes about your verbal and nonverbal communication. The practitioner will be careful not to compare you with another patient, as each individual is unique. The doctor will record his or her observations of you as well as your complaints and concerns and will most likely ask questions to better individualize the case. If you are seeking help for an acute illness, the doctor probably will focus on symptoms and feelings that have changed since you became ill. If you are complaining of a chronic ailment, the doctor will want to know as much as possible about your life and history. Conventional diagnostic testing can be useful in certain cases, but the alternative doctor's practice of "taking the case" allows him or her to get at the deeper source of your problem, rather than just treating your symptoms.

Natural medicine operates on Hippocrates' theory of *primum non nocere,* or "first do no harm." The goal is to treat illness with noninvasive, harmless remedies that invoke the body's innate healing powers. Natural medicine involves a comprehensive view of health, illness, treatment, and cure that meets the need of each individual person and helps to restore and maintain balance of the body and mind.

In some cases, natural treatment can suffice to cure an illness, but at other times allopathic treatments are required. If this is the case, alternative treatments can still be used to enhance the effectiveness of allopathic medicine, providing maximum healing for the individual. Healthy individuals also can pursue natural medicine regimens to maintain and enhance their physical, emotional, and mental well-being.

HISTORY OF NATURAL MEDICINE IN THE WEST

The word *naturopathy* was not used until the late nineteenth century, although its philosophy originated with Hippocrates, whose school of medicine existed around 400 B.C. Earlier people believed that disease was caused by supernatural powers. Hippocrates devised the theory that everything natural had a rational basis and that the causes of disease could be found in natural elements, such as air, water, or food. He also believed in *vis medicatrix naturae,* or the healing power of nature, and that the body had its own ability to heal itself.

The years from 1780 to 1850 marked the Age of Heroic Medicine. During this time, "heroic" treatments, such as bleeding, intestinal purgings, and blistering of the skin, were used to cure patients of their ills. These treatments were painful and harmful, and they often made patients worse, or even induced death. It was believed that bleeding, accomplished by lancing a vein or using leeches, removed impurities from the body. Intestinal purgings were performed by using mercuric chloride, which today we know causes severe metal poisoning; vomiting was induced by using other poisonous substances. The Age of Heroic Medicine was male-dominated and elitist, excluding women and nonconventional doctors. Some physicians who opposed heroic medicine practiced alternatives such as herbalism.

In 1810, a German doctor named Samuel Hahnemann (1755–1843) became disenchanted with the standard medicine of his day and began the practice of homeopathy. *Homeopathy* is derived from two Greek roots meaning "similar" and "disease, suffering." It is a philosophy of health and cure that is based on the principle that like cures like. That is, natural substances that produce particular symptoms in a healthy person can cure a sick person with those same symptoms.

Hahnemann did not actually originate the philosophy that like cures like; Hippocrates and others also had explored this concept previously. However, he did develop the theory into a viable alternative medical practice, homeopathy, which is discussed in greater detail in Chapter 3.

When Hahnemann died at the age of eighty-eight in 1843, he had many followers in Europe. The first homeopathic doctor came to the United States in 1828. In 1836, the Hahnemann Medical College opened in Philadelphia, and the first national medical society, the American Institute of Homeopathy, was established in 1844. As people began to react against heroic medical practices and politics, the Popular Health Movement was formed. It called for the repeal of all medical licensing laws, which was achieved by the end of the 1840s. This allowed physicians to practice whatever form of medicine they believed in. It was in this atmosphere that homeopathy flourished in the United States and set the stage for other alternative medicines, such as naturopathy, to take root.

Realizing that they were losing their foothold, the allopaths organized the American Medical Association (AMA) in 1846. While attacking homeopathy, they tried to give allopathy a more positive definition by claiming the word was based on German roots meaning "all therapies." Allopathy thus began to allow that a variety of remedies could be effective in treating a disease. The AMA required state medical societies to expel homeopaths and alternative healers, and in the 1860s, charges often were brought against allopaths who associated with these doctors. Allopaths began to wrest control of city hospitals and boards of health, and they succeeded in reestablishing licensing laws in all states. As the Popular Health Movement dissolved, alternative healers virtually were driven out of practice and denied any political influence.

By the 1880s, the homeopathic movement was being destroyed not only by the AMA but by its own internal philosophical divisions. Two groups of homeopaths emerged: those who were pure homeopaths, called Hahnemannians, and a larger, more modern group that included allopathic practices in their own work and that wanted to work with allopathic doctors rather than against them.

Dr. John Scheel of New York City coined the word *naturopathy* in 1895 to denote "nature cure." The earliest forms of natural treatments and preventions included good hygiene and hydrotherapy. Naturopathy began to be pursued in full force in the United States in 1902 by Benedict

Lust, who had emigrated from Germany in 1892. He had grown dissatisfied with conventional medicine and was intrigued by the European health spas, especially their treatment involving water cures and fasts. By the end of the nineteenth century, water cure was recognized as a vital healing therapy and referred to by the term *hydrotherapy*.

Lust intended to practice and teach hydrotherapy in the United States. Soon, however, his followers broadened their practices and healing philosophy to include an array of modalities, such as nutritional therapy, herbal medicine, homeopathy, spinal manipulation, exercise, hydrotherapy, electrotherapy, and stress management. Lust believed that in order to achieve good health, people should eliminate excessive consumption of toxic substances (such as caffeine, drugs, and alcohol), exercise, strive for a good mental attitude, and amend their lifestyles to include natural remedies such as fasting, proper diet, hydrotherapy, mud baths, chiropractic, and the like. He opened the American School of Naturopathy in New York City, which graduated its first class in 1902.

Natural medicine became very popular in the United States in the early twentieth century until the mid-1930s. At that point, conventional medicine again began to rise to prominence and popularity because of several factors. First, chemical and drug industries, which benefit more economically from allopathic than natural medicine, financially supported foundations that subsidized conventional medical schools. Second, orthodox medicine began to use less harmful treatments, and advances in health-care technology, particularly in surgery, convinced the public that conventional medicine was superior to natural medicine. The orthodox medical arena again began passing legislation that either limited or prohibited alternative health-care systems from flourishing.

Within the past two decades, since the 1970s, natural

medicine has begun to take hold again. Realizing that allopathic medicine may not have all of the answers or cures for their ills, people are seeking alternative treatments. As people begin to recognize the devastating contaminating effects of some technology on air, water, and food, they are also beginning to take action against such harmful practices. Finally, as the connection between the mind and body becomes ever more apparent, people are willing to make major lifestyle changes in order to protect and maintain their sense of physical and emotional balance. This is what natural medicine is all about and it is why more and more people are realizing the long-term benefits of alternative medical treatments.

LOCATING A
NATURAL MEDICINE
PRACTITIONER

One of the best ways to find a good alternative practitioner is to be referred by one of his or her patients, though you might not be fortunate enough to find one in this way. At the end of this book is a list of Natural Medicine Resources. Contact the listed organizations. Often they can make referrals to practitioners in your area, or they may have membership directories available.

When consulting a practitioner, interview him or her to learn as much as you can about the person and his or her practice. As a result of the interview, you will feel more comfortable seeking help from this person if you decide to do so, and that level of trust and comfort will facilitate a beneficial outcome for your treatment. The American Holistic Medical Association can send you a publication, *How to Choose a Holistic Health Practitioner*. The organization's address is listed in the Natural Medicine Resources section.

Following are some questions to ask a practitioner you interview:

- What schools did you attend and what is the extent of your training?
- What licenses or certificates do you hold?
- How long have you been in practice?
- What are your diagnostic and treatment procedures?
- What are the fees involved? What is the length of treatment or number of sessions proposed?
- Have you written any articles or books? (If so, they may be worth reading.)

CHAPTER THREE

Natural Therapies: An Overview

ORIENTAL MEDICINE

Oriental medicine defines health not as an absence of disease, as in Western medicine, but as a total state of well-being. It requires that the body be free from physical pain, but also encompasses the totality of the individual's thoughts, emotions, and beliefs. Health, in Eastern philosophy, is a state of mind and a way of life. Illness results from going against the natural laws of Heaven and Earth.

Oriental medicine began at least three thousand years ago, and has developed progressively as a science since approximately A.D. 200. It continues to flourish in the Eastern countries today, and many aspects of Oriental medicine are beginning to gain popularity as alternative treatments in the West. Oriental medicine involves several healing therapies, including acupuncture, herbs, nutrition, exercise (such as tai chi chuan and other martial arts), massage, and manipulation.

Taoism, Confucianism, and Buddhism are the underlying philosophies of Chinese medicine. According to Taoism, health reflects a harmony in Heaven, which is achieved through the balance of external and internal forces. A unity exists within the diversity of nature—a universal energy that exists in all things. This energy, called *chi*, is very difficult to describe. It has been explained as matter on the verge of becoming energy, while at the same time it is also energy on the verge of becoming matter. Everything in the universe is a result of the never-ending condensation of *chi* into matter and dispersion of *chi* into energy. In terms of Chinese medicine, *chi* needs to be understood in two ways. First, it nourishes the mind and body and has been described as the life force. Second, *chi* is produced by and indicates the function of the various *zang/fu,* or "spheres of function." *Zang/fu* refers not to a specific organ, such as the liver, but to the totality of body functions associated with the liver. Stomach *chi,* therefore, refers to various stomach functions, such as the transportation of food essences. The Chinese believe that *chi* flows throughout the human body. Health reflects a free flow of *chi,* but if the energy is imbalanced—if there is a blockage, an excess, or a deficiency of *chi* in specific body parts or organs—disease and illness occur.

Taoism also recognizes two opposite yet complementary qualities to all aspects of physical being. The philosophy derives from the notion that the universe was originally a ball of *chi* surrounded by chaos. When this mass of energy finally settled, it divided into the two opposing yet complementary qualities called *yin* and *yang.* Yin represents qualities that are negative, contractive, dark, small, of the right side, interior, of the nature of Earth. Yang, in contrast, is positive, expansive, light, big, of the left side, surface, of the nature of Heaven. All objects, animals, peoples, times, and places are a combination of yin and yang. It is believed that people are born with perfect yin and yang balance that is later thrown off kilter. Chinese doctors designate certain organs as being either of yin or yang qualities, and so are the foods and medicinal herbs that would be used to treat ailments of these organs.

Practitioners of Chinese medicine and philosophers believe in a dynamic cycle of evolution known as the five-element theory. All things are classified according to the five elements of wood, fire, earth, metal, and water. The body's organs are also characterized by the five elements; for example, the spleen and stomach are of the earth, and the lung and large intestine are of metal. These five elements are in a state of constant change and interact with one another. Doctors believe that organs affect other organs according to the elements. For instance, wood generates fire; therefore, the activity of the liver, which is characterized by wood, generates the activity of the heart, which is a fire organ. The relationships between the elements show doctors the direction in which *chi* flows within the body.

Just as the Chinese views about health differ from Western notions, so do their ideas about human anatomy. Chinese doctors identify twelve organs, or the *zang/fu*, which do not correspond directly to organs as we know them. Remember that *zang/fu* refers not to a specific organ, but to all of the body functions associated with that organ. This way of looking at the body probably evolved because ancient Chinese tradition prohibited the opening of corpses. Therefore, rather than developing a more detailed, concrete knowledge of anatomy, scientists and doctors focused on body functions instead of specific organs. The result is a more holistic understanding of function that embraces physical, mental, and emotional aspects.

Chinese medicine requires that the flow of *chi* in the body be influenced or moved, either by the practitioner or by the patient, so as to restore its balance. The flow of *chi* can be impeded by poor nutrition; lack of exercise; mental stress; fatigue; bad posture and breathing; pollution; physical growths such as tumors; or trauma, including those that result in scar tissue. A deficiency in *chi* can cause fatigue, depression, and various physical ailments. Excess *chi* might be responsible for hypertension, migraine headaches, or some types of arthritis. If the natural flow of *chi* through the body is altered in any way, a host of ailments could occur.

Chi flows through the body in fourteen pathways called meridians. The geography of the human body, as viewed by Eastern doctors, is based on these pathways as well as the *zang/fu* (organs) and bowels, and is very different from Western concepts of anatomy and physiology. Twelve of the meridians pass through a major organ and are linked to other meridians, so that all body parts have access to *chi.*

Practitioners of Oriental medicine examine and diagnose their patients in a way that is quite different from the quick, routine examinations and consultations patients in the West are accustomed to. There is careful questioning and observation of the patient, as well as monitoring of the patient's pulse. This is not pulse-checking as we know it, however. Rather, it is a fine art of detecting several layers of pulses in order to determine which body spheres are suffering. The doctor will take a pulse using the first three fingers of his or her hand, checking the patient's wrists with both light and firm pressure. The doctor will also identify pulses under each finger at both pressure levels—a total of six pulses for each wrist. Each pulse correlates with a specific body function sphere.

Acupuncture

One of the major Oriental healing arts is acupuncture, which involves the insertion of needles at specific points on the body. These special points are located along the various meridians, twelve of which correspond to a particular organ. It is indeed an art as well as a science to be able to locate the precise point at which a needle should be in-

serted. If it is not placed in the right position, the procedure will not have the desired effect. The purpose of acupuncture is to move or restore the flow of *chi* through the
insertion of the needles along the meridians relevant to the
illness.

The needles are inserted quickly and left in place for
several minutes. Sometimes the doctor will just pierce the
skin, while other times the needle will be inserted up to an
inch deep. The doctor might twirl the needle to increase
stimulation. Another process of stimulating the acupuncture points is called *moxabustion*. In one method of moxabustion, the needles' heads are wrapped with dry *moxa*
(Chinese wormwood) and burned. The needle conducts the
heat into the acupuncture point. In yet another process,
called electroacupuncture, the doctor connects each needle
to a small machine that stimulates the needles with a low
electrical pulse.

To those people raised with Western medical treatments, acupuncture is often viewed as a superstitious practice. The thought of having needles inserted into various
regions of the body, even places as delicate as the face, can
make even the staunchest Westerner squeamish. Those
who have experienced acupuncture, however, claim that it
is a painless, effective treatment for many illnesses. An acupuncture patient probably will feel a slight sensation when
the needles are inserted. As the acupuncture works, the
patient also might feel the presence of *chi* at the sites of the
needles or the movement of *chi* in the body.

All this discussion about *chi* and influencing its movement through the body may be difficult for you to accept.
Western scientists and doctors have devised several theories to explain why acupuncture works, especially when it is
used to alleviate pain. One theory is based on the fact that
the body produces endorphins and enkephalins, natural
painkilling chemicals that also can help allergies and de-

pression and can facilitate healing. Stimulating acupuncture points increases the body's production of endorphins and enkephalins. Another theory to explain acupuncture is that it has a placebo effect if the patient truly believes that it will help. Still another is based on the fact that some scientists and doctors feel that our vital energy is not *chi*, as the Chinese know it, but rather electricity. Acupuncture affects the way electricity travels along the meridians. Kirlian photography, which illustrates bioelectricity, provides evidence that this is a viable theory. The picture of a hand before and after acupuncture reveals an increased flow of electricity after the treatment. Finally, the gate theory of pain also is used to explain acupuncture. According to this theory, the body contains neuropathway "gates" along the spinal cord leading to the brain. Acupuncture closes the gates so that messages of pain do not reach the brain.

From a Chinese medicine point of view, acupuncture works as a result of regulating the flow of *chi* and blood. There is a Chinese expression, "There is no pain if there is free flow; if there is pain, there is no free flow."

Acupuncture has been shown to be an effective analgesic and has even been used instead of anesthetics during surgery. The stimulation of the acupuncture points in order to produce an analgesic effect causes the brain to release endorphins, which are the body's natural painkilling chemicals. Although Chinese doctors might use anesthetics during an operation, using acupuncture as an analgesic necessitates using only a fraction of the dose that a surgical patient in the West would receive. This is especially important for people who are sensitive to painkillers and anesthesia, as acupuncture is a harmless, safe way to treat pain.

Acupuncture can be an effective treatment for both terminal and nonterminal illnesses. It is a therapy that can be used alone or in combination with another treatment. For instance, if you are prone to back problems, you might want to consult a chiropractor who can help relieve pain and restore normal flow of energy.

Finding an Acupuncturist

If you are considering acupuncture as a healing therapy, try to get a referral from an acupuncture society or school, from the pain clinic at your local hospital, or from someone who has experienced the treatment firsthand. Investigate the training and experience of the doctor until you are satisfied with his or her qualifications. Licensing varies by state: Some license independent practitioners, while others restrict practice to medical doctors (those with an M.D. degree) or allow acupuncturists to work only under such a doctor's supervision. Contact the American Association of Acupuncture and Oriental Medicine, the National Commission for the Certification of Acupuncturists, or the National Accreditation Commission for Schools and Colleges of Acupuncture and Oriental Medicine (see the Natural Medicine Resources section) for information regarding licensing requirements in your state and for more information about acupuncture.

Visits to an acupuncturist range in cost from $35 to $75. Some insurance companies do cover the cost of acupuncture, but many still do not, and some will cover only those treatments recommended by a conventional doctor. Be sure to check your policy regarding your coverage for acupuncture.

When you visit an acupuncturist, make sure that the doctor uses either presterilized disposable needles or an autoclave, which is a sterilizing machine. An autoclave is the only effective way to sterilize needles and other medical or dental instruments sufficiently.

Typical Acupuncture Session

The exact details of a session with an acupuncturist will vary according to the training and philosophy of the therapist. A practitioner trained in traditional Chinese medicine will use acupuncture as part of a total treatment regimen and will offer a course of healing quite different from an American medical doctor trained in using acupuncture as symptomatic first aid. Even among acupuncturists, there are significant variations in style and approach. Someone trained in traditional Chinese medicine will practice differently from someone trained in Japanese, Korean, or French acupuncture. However, some general observations can be made about a typical acupuncture session for the chronic pain patient.

The session will start with a diagnosis or assessment of your symptoms or complaints. The therapist may look at the color of your face and the condition of your tongue, skin, eyes, fingernails, and hair. He or she may ask for a urine or stool sample to check its color.

Next, the practitioner will ask you questions. He or she may want to know about your appetite, your body fluid secretions, and your individual and family medical history.

Finally, the acupuncturist may palpate your back, chest and abdomen and take your pulse, both important techniques for determining the condition of your body-energy flow. This is similar to the pulse reading your doctor or nurse performs, except the acupuncturist will check three places from each wrist and three depths of flow at each place. This gives the acupuncturist a sense of the flow and balance of your body energy and the location of any blockage or deficiency. With the information gathered from the interview and pulse reading, the acupuncturist will determine your specific imbalance and the point or points of needling that will be appropriate treatment.

At this point the acupuncturist has a good idea of your condition and needs. You can now get some answers to your questions: What kind of pain relief can I realistically expect from acupuncture? What's the probability of long-term relief? Although, as in all natural sciences, exact guaranteed answers are not possible, an experienced acupuncturist should be able to give you some insight into your prognosis for change.

Now the acupuncturist is ready to insert the needles. One practitioner may needle a patient in two spots for thirty seconds while another might find it necessary to use ten needles for twenty minutes on that same patient. The range of treatment techniques is quite vast. However, in general, you can expect your treatment to last about twenty minutes with needles in place.

Acupuncture is not painful. You'll feel a slight pricking sensation as the needles are inserted into the skin. Then you'll feel a second sensation when your body energy comes in contact with the needles; this may be a feeling of warmth, dullness, an ache, or even a feeling like a slight electrical shock.

Often acupuncture works to relieve pain in a gradual rather than a dramatic manner. After your first visit, you should not expect to go home completely pain free. You may feel some change in the intensity of your pain, but readjusting the body's energy flow so the body can better heal itself is a process that occurs over time. However, with acute muscle sprains and strains, the pain relief is often dramatic.

At the second and subsequent treatment sessions the acupuncturist will reevaluate your status. He or she will repeat the physical exam and talk to you about your pain experience. The therapist will want to know if you've noticed any changes in the way you feel your pain. Is it more bearable? Has the intensity diminished? Are you incapacitated less frequently? In addition, he or she will want to know about other changes in the physical, emotional or mental spheres. Based on the exam and this information, the acupuncturist will either repeat or alter the needling process of the previous visit.

Acupuncture for chronic pain relief is not a remedy that must be continued for the rest of your life. Your acupuncturist should be able to give you an idea of how long it will take to resolve the imbalance that is intensifying your pain. However, if after ten to twelve visits you see no change in your pain or other symptoms, you should discuss this with your acupuncturist to determine whether acupuncture is an appropriate therapy.

Acupressure

Acupressure is a therapy that is similar to acupuncture in that it uses the same geography of meridians and acupuncture (or acupressure) points. Instead of using needles, however, the practitioner uses hands or feet to gently pressure the appropriate points. Acupressure relaxes tense muscles, improves blood circulation, and stimulates the body's ability to heal itself.

Acupressure, which predates acupuncture, was developed approximately five thousand years ago by the Chinese. They discovered that pressing certain points on the body not only relieved localized pain but could affect other parts of the body and internal organs as well. Acupressure was increasingly disregarded, however, as the Chinese began to use needles to stimulate the acupressure points.

Acupressure points are illustrated on pages 321–324 at the back of the book. The descriptions of treatments for various conditions will refer to these diagrams and name the corresponding numbers that are relevant to use. For example, in treating migraine headaches, the text will read:

"GB20, located below the base of the skull in the hollows between the vertical neck muscles." Once you locate the point on yourself or the person you are treating, apply firm and steady pressure. It will take practice and experimentation to find the points and pressure that work for you.

Acupressure is not intended to cure serious illness or replace orthodox medical treatments for those illnesses. It can, however, increase relaxation, improve circulation, and ease pain, thereby maximizing health. Since it utilizes the same points as in acupuncture, specific *chi* or blood regulating or nourishing benefits associated with the points can be realized. It is an inexpensive and simple therapy to learn and one that, if practiced correctly, is entirely safe. Here are some tips to bear in mind when administering acupressure to yourself or others:

- Use only gentle pressure; it should not cause any pain.
- Since there are a number of acupoints that are forbidden during pregnancy, you should work on a pregnant woman only under the instruction of a qualified acupuncture or acupressure practitioner.
- Do not use acupressure on someone who is taking drugs or alcohol.
- Do not administer acupressure immediately after eating.
- It is best for the patient to sit or lie down, as he or she may feel drowsy during a procedure.

Acupressure and Pain Relief

Acupressure can be used to maintain the body's balance of energy, maintain well-being, and treat the symptoms of chronic pain in much the same way as acupuncture. By maintaining a free and balanced flow of *chi* and blood, there will be no pain. It is possible that pressure applied to acupoints can close the gate at the base of the spine, thus blocking pain signals. The pressure also may stimulate the brain to release endorphins, the body's natural painkillers. Once the pain message is interrupted, muscles relax and blood, lymph, and oxygen can flow more easily into the affected area. This in turn allows for more nutrients to reach the affected areas and for toxins to be carried away, thereby increasing immunity and promoting health.

Also, we know that tension and stress can cause neuro-muscular imbalances that can flare up into painful conditions. By relieving tension and increasing circulation, acupressure reduces and even prevents pain, while at the same time promoting relaxation and healing.

Because it stimulates the release of endorphins and relaxes muscular tension, acupressure can be an effective therapy for all kinds of pain. From toothaches, earaches, and backaches to the pain of cancer and old age, acupressure can be an effective adjunct to a complete pain-relief program.

Actually, acupressure is a broad term for a number of massage therapies that use the body meridians to promote good health. The following are four of the better-known forms of acupressure.

Acupressure first aid: Acupressure can be used for the temporary relief of specific physical problems.

Jin Shin: At key acupuncture points on selected meridians and channels, Jin Shin uses a pattern of gentle prolonged point-holding. Points are held for one to five minutes. Jin Shin Jyutsu, Jin Shin Jitsu, and Jin Shin Do are all forms of Jin Shin.

Shiatsu: In Japanese, *shiatsu* literally means (*shi*) finger (*atsu*) pressure. This technique uses a rhythmic series of finger pressure, stretching and tapping along the body meridians. Points are held only three to five seconds.

Tui Na: Tui Na is Chinese massage that stimulates the acupressure points, using a wide variety of hand movements.

Finding an Acupressurist

Finding a competent acupressurist is a bit more difficult than finding an acupuncturist because there are no state licensing laws for the training, certification, or administration of this form of natural medicine. However, each type of acupressure (Jin Shin, Tui Na, shiatsu, and so on) has a governing organization that provides training and certification by that group. It is best to locate a practitioner through such an organization or school of training.

A Typical Acupressure Session

The details of an acupressure session will vary according to the type of massage being applied. Each style is different in the patterns of point-holding, the number of points held, the length of time each point is pressed or held, the pressure used, and the technique of applying that pressure. However, while the specific techniques of acupressure differ, the goals are the same: to balance the flow of energy in the body and stimulate its recuperative powers.

In some ways, a session with a professional acupressurist will be similar to a visit to an acupuncturist. The therapist will first assess your health and needs. This may be done by talking about your medical history, past therapies, medications, and present needs. The acupressurist may then use any one of the traditional assessment techniques, which include pulse diagnosis, face reading, and tongue or skin examination.

The acupressure session can be conducted in a variety of settings and postures. You may be asked to sit in a chair or on a stool, or you may lie on a padded table or on a carpeted floor. Although a quiet, relaxed atmosphere is most desirable, acupressure can be administered almost anywhere.

An acupressure session generally passes through two or three stages. First there is a general energy balancing, followed by specific attention to the blocked meridians that are at the root of the imbalance. Finally, many practitioners add some sort of a technique to bring the session to a close.

Movement and Meditation

Advocates of Oriental medicine also believe that you can heal yourself through the dedicated practice of different kinds of movement and meditation.

The martial arts are different forms of exercise that require and develop supreme control, discipline, and strength in the individual. A gentle martial art, tai chi chuan, can help a person develop inner strength and control. The Chinese believe that movement is essential for the human body. Tai chi chuan involves slow, deliberate movements, a sense of communion with nature, and concentration on finding one's *chi*. The philosophy is that if one can locate one's *chi* and learn how to use it, one can maintain good health. Some martial arts schools offer classes in tai chi chuan, and it is an exercise that requires many years of dedicated practice to develop fully.

Another form of meditation, called chi-gong, is also used

to find one's *chi*. Chinese doctors believe that a ball of *chi* is located in the abdominal or pelvic region, and through meditation people can learn to move their *chi* to the appropriate areas of their body. The idea, again, is to learn to influence the flow of *chi* so as to maintain its balance in the body.

Even when you are working with a doctor or trying to heal yourself, all Oriental medicine seems to require willing and dedicated participation on your part. Oriental medicine has been practiced for thousands of years, and it is effective. Of course, as with any healing treatment, not all forms will work in every case or all of the time. Oriental medicine does seem to substantiate, however, the connection of the mental and physical. This belief is inherent in the Eastern philosophy of health, and it is utilized to treat illness and to maximize health.

HOMEOPATHY

Homeopathy is a system of health care and treatment that was developed in the 1800s by Dr. Samuel Hahnemann. The philosophy of homeopathy is holistic, viewing the individual as a totality of interdependent parts and working from the notion that the mental and physical realms are inseparable. Hahnemann believed that orthodox medicine was a system of "contraries," meaning that doctors treated the symptoms of an illness by using drugs that oppose, or suppress, them. He began to call conventional medicine *allopathic*, meaning "different" and "disease, suffering." Hahnemann recognized that removing or masking symptoms did not treat the underlying cause of the illness, which could, in effect, develop into a more serious condition.

In homeopathy, symptoms are seen as a healthy response of the body's defense mechanism. The vital force, or vital energy, acts to keep the body in balance. When the body is threatened by some harmful external influence, the vital force (or defense mechanism) produces symptoms in its struggle against the harmful agent. Therefore, to a homeopathic doctor, fever is a sign that the body is fighting illness. A cough, which an allopathic doctor would try to suppress with medication, is seen by the homeopath as the natural way to expel mucus from the body. Bear in mind that this does not mean you must suffer with coughing all day long. You can use herbal cough drops and drink teas with honey, for example, to soothe your throat. However, if you are not willing to endure some discomfort during your sickness, you should reassess whether natural medicine treatments are appropriate for you.

Believing that drug prescriptions for specific illnesses often were based on an inadequate understanding of the drugs and their effects, Hahnemann began to test, or "prove," drugs on healthy women and men, including himself, to determine their effects. He tested remedies on people rather than animals because he knew that people usually react differently than animals do. This human testing is possible because the homeopathic remedies are nontoxic. In more than two hundred years of using the homeopathic formulations, there has been no reported case of a permanent adverse reaction.

In his provings, Hahnemann discovered that each remedy induced particular symptoms in a healthy person. When that remedy was given to a sick person exhibiting those same symptoms, it helped cure the person. Based on this notion that like cures like, Hahnemann formulated the Law of Similars. It states that a substance causing certain symptoms in a healthy person can cure a sick person with the same symptoms. The theory behind the Law of Similars is that the body enlists its own energies to heal itself and defend against illness. If a substance that causes a similar response in terms of similar symptoms is administered, the body steps up its fight against it, thereby promoting cure.

In an attempt to lessen the initial aggravating effects that remedies sometimes had on patients, Hahnemann administered very small dosages. Ironically, he discovered that the smaller the dose, the more powerful the effect. This led him to develop the Law of Infinitesimals, which states that the smaller the dose, the more effective it is in stimulating the body to respond against the illness.

In order to prepare smaller and smaller doses, Hahnemann would put a substance through a series of dilutions. He would begin with the original substance, putting one part in nine parts of an 87 percent solution of alcohol and distilled water. He then subjected to *succussion,* or vigorously agitated, the vial by striking it one hundred times against a leather pad. Hahnemann believed that subjecting the substance to succussion activated the therapeutic potential of it. This first step yields a one-in-ten dilution, also indicated as a "1× dilution." Hahnemann would then take one part of this 1× dilution and put it in nine parts of diluent, subjecting it to succussion to yield a 2× dilution. This process, referred to as the Law of Potentization, could continue indefinitely, producing increasingly potent dosages.

Hahnemann believed in administering one homeopathic remedy at a time in order to establish its effects. He treated all patients as whole people, taking their symptoms as part of their whole being rather than treating them separately, and apart from the rest of the person. This method differs from orthodox medicine in which specialists treat specific illnesses and body parts, and patients often take many drugs simultaneously.

Homeopathy views health as a state of freedom and well-being on three interdependent levels: physical, emotional, and mental. The most serious symptoms usually affect the deeper parts of a person; therefore, it is most important to treat the mental state, then the emotional, and finally the physical. This is in keeping with the holistic view of natural medicine, which treats the entire person—physically and mentally. In other words, a homeopath would say that it is not enough to treat you for migraine headaches, because if the stressors producing the migraines are not addressed, the migraines will recur or other symptoms could develop.

The German homeopath, Constantine Hering, who emigrated to the United States in the 1830s, recorded the changes in posttreatment symptoms. Based on his findings that healing occurs from the inside out, he laid the groundwork for Hering's Law of Cure, which is recognized not only by homeopaths but by acupuncturists and psychotherapists as well.

Hering's Law states that cure occurs from within outward, from the most vital to the least important organs. The body deals with the most significant aspect of the condition first, shifting during treatment to the next most important aspect, and so on. For instance, healing is believed to be in progress—from the inside out—if your chest pains subside but a skin rash develops. During homeopathic treatment, your condition can change so that the same or other remedies may be needed to facilitate the entire process of cure.

Hering's Law further states that symptoms will appear and disappear in the reverse order in which they originally appeared. The patient may also reexperience symptoms from a past condition. According to Hering, healing often begins with the upper body parts and descends. Therefore, if chronic headaches subside but stiff fingers are felt, the homeopath might believe that healing is taking place, and gradually the fingers should return to normal. At times, healing may not follow the traditional pattern of Hering's

Law, but as long as the patient feels stronger and is improved overall, it is safe to assume that the treatment is working.

Based on the order "first, do no harm," homeopathy is a safe and effective system of treating many common acute and chronic ailments. For a temporary, minor, self-limited illness or injury, you probably can treat yourself with homeopathic remedies after consulting with your doctor. You can obtain remedies from homeopathic pharmacists, or even from some drugstores or health-food stores. For a more chronic, persistent illness, you should consult a qualified homeopathic practitioner. Professional homeopathic medical doctors graduate from conventional four-year medical schools with a Doctor of Medicine (M.D.) degree and often complete postgraduate training in homeopathy to learn this holistic specialty. Homeopathic schools can be found worldwide, but to master the art and science of the system, physicians often learn from experienced homeopathic doctors. The fees charged by homeopaths vary, as does insurance coverage. Some states and insurance companies honor homeopathic treatment and some do not, and some will cover it only if it is performed by a licensed medical doctor.

HYDROTHERAPY

Sometimes the most obvious and simplest remedies are the ones most often overlooked. Consider water—it composes two-thirds of our bodies and covers four-fifths of the earth's surface. Human beings can survive for weeks without food but only a few days without water. How can an element so common and abundant possibly be useful in healing?

The use that probably comes to mind first is the practice

of swimming as physical therapy or bathing in a whirlpool to soothe sore muscles. But water has other healthful benefits as well, and in its various forms it can even be used to treat injuries and illnesses. It can work on the whole body, as in a bath, or on one area, as in the use of a compress. Water benefits the entire body by reenergizing it. Using a water therapy on one body part can also affect another beneficially, such as the use of a hot footbath to aid decongestion. Every organ and cell requires water, which helps nourish, detoxify, and maintain the right temperature of the body.

One of the earliest records of the therapeutic use of water dates back to the Greek god of medicine known as Aesculapius. At his temples, bathing and massage were used as a form of cure. Hippocrates also used water therapeutically. He advocated drinking water to alleviate fever, and he believed that baths could fight sickness. The Greek doctor Galen, who wrote Rome's outstanding medical text, also believed baths, both hot and cold, had beneficial effects, as did the Greek medical writer Celsus. Of course, this is true, because, in fact, one of the major reasons that health has increased over the ages is that sanitation and hygiene have improved.

In the eighteenth century, German, English, and Italian clergy revived the therapeutic use of water. In 1797, a Scottish doctor, James Currie, wrote a book called *Medical Reports on the Effects of Water, Cold and Warm, as a Remedy in Fever and Febrile Diseases*. In the early nineteenth century, Vincent Preissnitz, a Silesian farmer, reinvented water therapy using methods such as dousings, showers, immersions, and single and double compresses. His procedures spread to England, Germany, and Scandinavia, as well as the United States.

Later in the nineteenth century, Sebastian Kniepp adapted Preissnitz's techniques into his own theories of hydrotherapy. Kniepp, born in Bavaria in 1821, was a frail and sickly person. After reading a pamphlet about water cures, he decided to plunge into an icy cold river in the middle of winter with the hope that it would cure his ailments. Kniepp jumped into the river every day, and although it might seem absurd, he claimed that over time he became physically stronger. Along with Preissnitz's techniques, Kniepp claimed that walking in cold water or on wet grass was therapeutic.

Hydrotherapy is based on the law of action and reaction. If the skin is heated, either by a hot bath or compress, blood is immediately drawn to the surface and then returns to the deeper blood vessels. Likewise, cold water will drive blood away from the surface, but will cause a secondary effect of warmth as the blood returns to the tissues and vessels from which it was pushed away. This concept of immediate action followed by a secondary and more lasting reaction is a basic principle of hydrotherapy.

The different forms and temperatures of water have different physical and chemical effects on the body. Cold water is essentially restorative and reenergizing. It can reduce fever, act as a diuretic and anesthetic, alleviate pain, help relieve constipation, and eliminate toxins from the body. Ice and ice water can relieve the pain of burns, help control bleeding, and reduce swelling from injury. Warm water, in contrast, has a relaxing effect. Hot baths induce perspiration, which is essential in eliminating toxins from the body. Hot compresses and baths can reduce pain and inflammation, although cold water should be used for inflammation due to injury. This is important because hot water increases blood flow and would thereby increase inflammation in an injury. Alternating hot and cold baths can help increase circulation. Steam is a form of hydrotherapy that opens pores, increases perspiration, and sometimes alleviates chest congestion. Humidifying air is good for those who suffer from sinus conditions and airborne allergies.

Water has therapeutic uses when used internally or externally, at varying degrees of temperatures and pressures, and in its three forms: ice, liquid, or steam. Ice can be used as an anesthetic to chill the skin and dull pain. Boiling water is an antiseptic that can cleanse food and clothing. Hot compresses placed on the abdomen and herbal teas can work as antispasmodics to relieve cramps. If you need a diuretic, try drinking ice water or herbal tea or applying a hot, moist compress on your lower back; these all cause the kidneys to increase urine production. Colon irrigation, enemas, genital irrigation, the drinking of water, the taking of a sauna or hot baths all help to eliminate toxins. Drinking an emetic, such as salt water, can induce vomiting in order to expel certain poisonous substances. Finally, hot or cold baths or showers, whirlpools, and salt baths have a stimulating effect, while warm showers or herbal baths can act as a sedative.

Many different types of water application are used in hydrotherapy. Local heat can be achieved with a moist, hot compress or hot-water bottle; local cold requires a cold compress, frozen bandage, or ice pack or bag. A cold double compress is a cold compress covered with a dry cloth, such as wool or flannel, which creates internal heat. A pack is a larger form of the double compress, or it can be a clay, mustard, or flaxseed poultice. Alcohol, water, or witch hazel can be used in sponging, and you can achieve tonic friction by rubbing with a sponge or washcloth. Therapeutic showers can alternate between hot and cold, and the pressure of the shower can vary. Steam is therapeutic too, from a sauna, vaporizer, or humidifier.

One of the most common and most appreciated hydrotherapy techniques is the bath, a total immersion of either the body or a part of the body, such as hands, feet, arms, eyes, or fingers. Depending on the ailment you wish to treat, baths can be cold, tepid, or hot, can be long or short in duration, and can involve massage using a sponge, bath mitten, or loofah brush to create tonic friction. Baths can consist of plain water or contain salts, herbs, oatmeal, or mud. Following is a list of bath additives and their therapeutic benefits:

Apple cider vinegar: Fights fatigue; relieves sunburn and itchy skin.

Borax/cornstarch/bicarbonate of soda: Good antiseptic.

Bran: Softens skin and relieves itchiness.

Chamomile: Soothes skin and opens pores; helps to relieve insomnia and digestive problems.

Dead Sea salts: Restores body after injury.

Epsom salts: Increases perspiration, relaxes muscles, and helps to relieve catarrh.

Fennel/nettle: Helps to rid skin of impurities.

Ginger powder: Relaxes muscles, tones skin, and increases circulation. (Use in small amounts as it is very powerful.)

Hayflower/oatstraw: Helps to rid skin of impurities.

Nutmeg: Increases perspiration.

Oatmeal: Good for skin problems, such as itchiness, hives, windburn, and sunburn.

Pine: Increases perspiration, softens skin, and relieves rashes.

Rosemary: Stimulates blood circulation.

Sage: Stimulates sweat glands.

Salt: Promotes a relaxing effect.

Sulfur: Good antiseptic and helps to rid skin of parasites; helps relieve acne.

It is easy and inexpensive to treat yourself to a wide variety of baths. Most of the listed herbs and preparations can be bought in drugstores, herbal pharmacies, health-food stores, or through catalogs. Remember to purchase them in small quantities since they lose their potency in approximately one year.

BOTANICAL MEDICINE

Botanical medicine, also referred to as herbalism, plant healing, physiomedicalism, medical herbalism, and phyto-therapy, uses remedies made from plants called herbs. Whereas botanists define herbs as any plants that do not contain woody fibers, medicinal herbalists define them as any plant that has healing properties. Herbal remedies can also come from trees, ferns, seaweeds, or lichens, and herbalists will use whole plants, rather than isolating the principal active compounds from them. Whole plants contain proteins, enzymes, vitamins, minerals, and other trace elements that readily assimilate in the body. In fact, the three fatty acids essential for life—linoleic, linolenic, and arachidonic—are all found in plants. Botanical medicine is a safe and natural way to treat specific ailments and assist recuperation from illness in order to restore physiological balance.

The history of botanical medicine goes back through the ages, with "recipes" for herbal remedies being passed from generation to generation. Plants are natural agents of cure, and animals have an instinct for their curative powers. You've probably seen a dog nibble on grass. No, he doesn't think he's part goat—but he might have a bellyache and is eating the grass to aid his digestion. For centuries, Native Americans have chewed willow-tree bark to cure headaches. The bark contains salicylic acid, the active ingredient in aspirin.

Traditional herbal medicine originated in ancient times in India, China, and Egypt, with the earliest records appearing in Egypt and Assyria. Many of the plants listed in these and in Greek documents are still used today. Over time, herbalists have compiled classifications—descriptions of plants arranged according to their medicinal properties. Today, there are more than 750,000 plants in the world, and only a small percentage have been evaluated. The World Health Organization investigates and supports herbal medicine throughout the world in order to learn more about this natural method of healing.

Plants are used not only in botanical medicine but in allopathic medicine as well, and once served as the basis for nearly all drugs. In order to appreciate the benefits of botanical medicine, it is useful to look at how allopathy has used plants in preparing drugs.

Until the 1800s, most drugs were given by mouth in the form of ground leaves, roots, or flowers, or in teas, tinctures, or extracts. Doctors studied botany as a matter of course, and herbalists without medical training, particularly women, also flourished.

Prior to the 1800s, there was no standard clinical evidence on which doctors could base their selection of drugs for treatment. In 1803, a German pharmacist isolated morphine from opium, signifying the first time that a pure active principle had been obtained from a crude plant drug. With this pure form of morphine, doctors could give exact doses, knowing their effects. In the mid-nineteenth century, there was a push to isolate pure forms of active principles from medicinal plants. By 1870, caffeine had been isolated from coffee, nicotine from tobacco, and cocaine from coca.

These isolated compounds are generally more toxic than the whole plants from which they are derived. Scientists and doctors believed it was better to treat patients with the purified drug, and they disregarded other compounds in the plant. Herbalists, however, recognized that the whole plant has a different effect from the isolated substance since it contains many other vital ingredients that interact to give an overall effect.

Besides using isolated principles, chemists also experiment with molecules to synthesize new drugs. Their goal usually is to increase the potency and efficacy of the drug. More potent drugs can be risky, however, given that doctors often prescribe numerous medications simultaneously. And some drugs are so potent as to be addictive. Adverse drug reactions, or side effects, are the most common kind of iatrogenic (doctor-caused) illness.

Many commonly used drugs are derived from plants. For instance, digitoxin comes from foxglove (*Digitalis purpurea*) and is prescribed for heart failure; atropine is from deadly nightshade (*Atropa belladonna*) and dilates pupils; morphine comes from the opium poppy (*Papaver somniferum*) and is a powerful painkiller.

Herbalists may use the root, rhizome, stem, leaf, flower, seed, fruit, bark, wood, resin, or whole plant in preparing an herbal medication. Familiar with the interactions of various plants, herbalists usually will use several plants or extracts in one preparation, since they can sometimes be more effective when combined than when used separately. Plants contain oils, alkaloids (nitrogen compounds), tannins, resins, fats, carbohydrates, proteins, and enzymes that all contribute to their medicinal action. Each substance has a function and can support, control, or otherwise affect the other constituents. In using the whole plant, the herbalist will get the most gentle, safe, and effective benefit from the treatment.

Herbal remedies can be taken in the form of tablets, capsules, lotions, ointments, suppositories, inhalants, or teas and juices. For herbal drinks, the basic proportion is 1 ounce (25 grams) of herbs to 1 pint (0.5 liter) of liquid. Herb teas will keep for three days in a tightly covered container in the refrigerator. Following is a list of common terms referring to botanical medications:

Carminative: Relieves flatulence, colic.

Cholagogue: Stimulates release of bile from the gallbladder.

Decoction: Drink made from roots, bark, or berries simmered in boiling water and strained.

Demulcent: Soothing substance for the skin.

Emmenagogue: Stimulates menstruation.

Emollient: Used internally to soothe membranes or externally to soften skin.

Infusion: Boiling water is poured over leaves, flowers, or the whole plant (excluding seeds and berries).

Nervine: That which is calming.

Ointments: Applied externally; effective for skin conditions.

Poultice: Crushed plant and hot water mixed to produce a paste that is wrapped in a thin cloth and applied to the skin.

Pressed juice: Juice from fresh plants is rich in vitamins and minerals; can be used in tinctures or diluted in water.

Teas: Made from pouring boiling water over fermented leaves or stalks from one or more plants;

fermentation produces tannin; premade teabags can be purchased.

Tinctures: One part herb in five parts of diluted alcohol.

Tisane: Add boiling water to fresh or dried plant, usually green leaves.

You can dry your own leaves by laying them on a wire rack in a warm, dry place for forty-eight hours; store in airtight glass containers. This should keep for one year. When preparing a tisane, use a separate pot from the one you use for tea, as tannin will interfere with the tisane remedy.

Vulnerary: Used to treat and heal wounds.

An herbalist can give you information as to appropriate herbs used to treat various symptoms. A consultation with an herbalist is similar to one with other natural healers. The herbalist will check your heart and pulse, physical symptoms, and perhaps perform some laboratory tests, such as blood and urine analyses. More important, the herbal practitioner will spend quite some time observing, talking, questioning, and listening to you in order to determine the imbalance and disharmony of your body and life.

If you find a satisfactory course of treatment with a particular herbalist, it is good to stay with that person so as not to disrupt the healing process. Sometimes symptoms are aggravated before healing occurs, and some people and certain disorders take longer to heal than others. Patience and willing participation in your treatment is essential in order to maximize the benefits of botanical medicine. And any herbal treatment should be undertaken only in consultation with your physician.

Botanical Medicine and Pain

A number of herbs have an analgesic effect and often are used in the treatment of chronic pain. Quite commonly, white willow bark *(Salix alba)* is recommended for any ailment or condition that is treated by conventional medicine with aspirin. The active ingredient of aspirin, salicylic, is derived from this source.

Other analgesic herbs include passion flower, hops, and valerian.

For chronic pain that stems from a condition involving inflammation, such as arthritis, migraine, or musculoskeletal pain, practitioners might recommend feverfew, which has anti-inflammatory properties.

The exact amount and the appropriate form of these herbs best suited to treat your condition depends on many considerations, such as the kind of pain and its intensity. You'll need the help of an herbalist or naturopath to choose what's best for you.

PHYSICAL MEDICINE

Chiropractic

The word *chiropractic* means "treatment by the hands, or manipulation." It is a system of healing that was developed by David Daniel Palmer (1845–1913) in Iowa in 1895. Palmer believed that displacements of the spine caused pressure on nerves, which created pain or symptoms in other parts of the body.

Although chiropractic medicine subscribes to traditional concepts of anatomy and physiology, it differs from traditional medicine in that it is holistic, meaning it considers the patient as a whole, with an emphasis on body structure.

Practitioners rely on X rays and standard orthopedic and neurological tests to diagnose problems, focusing on abnormalities of the spine. Treatment often involves direct thrust on specific vertebrae that are out of alignment, which helps to restore the flow of energy. Two terms that you will encounter in chiropractic are *adjustment* and *manipulation*. Adjustments involve dynamic thrusts (rapid, precise, and painless force) to a specific vertebra in order to remove any interference with nerves. It is not only the adjustment itself that is important, but the body's healing reaction to it. Manipulations are more general reorderings of bones to realign joints and increase the patient's range of motion.

Chiropractic is helpful in treating many conditions, including back pain and musculoskeletal disorders as well as certain systemic illnesses, such as asthma, migraines, and digestive problems. These systemic disorders, however, can be helped only if there is evidence of a structural and neurological involvement. Chiropractic treatment must be administered by a qualified and licensed professional, and it usually involves multiple visits in order to maintain proper spinal alignment. Initial visits can run from $50 to $150, with routine visits priced at approximately $50, and most insurance companies do provide coverage for this treatment. Chiropractors usually undergo at least two years of college plus an additional four years of professional education, and they must pass state and national licensing examinations.

Chiropractic Medicine for the Treatment of Pain

Chiropractic treatment of chronic pain is a highly effective remedy that's considered "natural" because of its noninvasive and sometimes nontraditional approach. Studies in North America, Europe, and Australia report that approximately 80 percent of chiropractic practice is for musculoskeletal pain, with low-back and neck pain the predominant presenting complaints. Another 10 percent is for headache and migraine.

Major pain-related problems treated with chiropractic medicine include:

1. Spinal and pelvic involvements: disk syndromes; low-back problems; cervical, thoracic, and lumbar strains; sprains; and subluxations

2. Spinosomatic syndromes: neuralgias arising in the spinal column and the pelvis but radiating into the arms and legs

3. General muscular ailments: fatigue and postural defects of the body (causing muscle pain in the back and neck), sprains and strains of the rib cage, traumatic bursitis or tendonitis of the shoulder or elbow

4. Spinal visceral syndromes: functional disorders of the internal organs and systems that are caused by irritation of nerve pathways

Finding a Chiropractor

Your decision as to what type of chiropractor to seek for treatment is a personal one based on your particular ailment and your personal needs. However, it is important to choose an experienced doctor through medical or personal recommendation. Chiropractic treatment involves highly specific adjustment of the spinal tissues. Always be certain that your chiropractor is state licensed and reputable. Never allow a "paraprofessional" or other untrained, unlicensed person attempt to manipulate your spine; this could worsen your problem rather than help.

Typical Chiropractic Session

Striving to treat the cause of the pain, not merely the symptom, all chiropractors are professionally trained in clinical diagnosis, clinical neurology, differential diagnosis, laboratory diagnosis, and the use of special instruments needed for regional diagnosis. To begin an evaluation and diagnosis, the practitioner will look for a structural problem such as subluxation, partially misaligned and mechanically dysfunctional vertebrae, and other joints that are off center. Of course, the chiropractor also looks for any pathologies that may be present. These disorders can negatively affect the healthy functioning of various tissues, organs, and systems of the body.

No responsible chiropractor will claim to *cure* organic disease such as ulcers, tumors, or shingles through the adjustment of the spine, but clinical experience and scientific studies suggest that pain originating in the spine plays an important role in many conditions. *The Chiropractic Report* of March 1993 notes that Kunert, a West German cardiologist prominent in the European manual medicine school in the 1950s and 1960s, has case examples of chiropractic aid where the medical diagnoses were respiratory block and heart disease. The primary causes were found in the alignment of the spinal cord and could be corrected by spinal manipulation. Following extensive clinical and research experience, Kunert concluded that "lesions of the spinal column . . . are perfectly capable of simulating, accentuating or making a major contribution to organic diseases. There can . . . be no doubt that the state of the spinal column does have a bearing on the functional status of the internal organs."

In addition, chiropractic medicine also can be used to prevent many types of disease. Maintaining the general good health of the body through spinal manipulation can help increase the strength of the immune system. By relaxing tense muscle fibers, the chiropractor improves circulation, allowing blood to flow freely and toxins to be released and eliminated. Increased circulation also brings more oxygen and other nutrients throughout the body, increasing the body's resistance to illness and promoting a stronger and healthier body system.

The chronic pain patient who visits a chiropractor will soon find that chiropractic treatment provides more than just temporary relief. There are emotional/mental benefits to be gained that give chiropractic an advantage over conventional medical practices. Some medical historians believe that for many, the turning point away from conventional medicine came with the advent of technical aids such as the stethoscope, which reduced the opportunities for human contact. As a hands-on methodology, chiropractic medicine instills a sense of comfort and relaxation. For you, the pain patient, this alone can relieve the anxiety, stress, and tension known to aggravate, intensify, and prolong pain.

Best of all, recent scientific studies have shown conclusively that chiropractic spinal treatment is not only an effective remedy in the majority of mechanical back and neck pain cases but also has long-term benefits as well. This alone positions modern chiropractors to be key players in treating nonsurgical back pain.

Over a hundred manipulative techniques are taught and practiced today. This makes a description of a typical session difficult because almost every chiropractor has a unique technique and program. There are, however, certain things you may expect from a chiropractor during treatment of chronic pain.

A typical visit may include a complete orthopedic, neurological, and postural examination to help diagnose which tissues are involved in the pain—i.e., disk, nerve, bone, ligament, and so on. Then, X rays of the afflicted site may be taken. From this, an exact diagnosis can be made and a treatment program may begin.

Some chiropractors administer treatment only during sessions without any type of comprehensive program, while others may prescribe an at-home program of remedies and supplements, such as rehabilitative exercises to strengthen weak muscles or correct posture, physiotherapy, hydrotherapy, heat treatments, braces, yoga, massage, or acupressure.

Massage

The word *massage* derives from both the Greek *masso* ("knead") and the Arabic *mass* ("press gently"). It is a form of physical medicine that is harmless, comfortable, and relaxing. While a massage can be given by anyone, a trained massage therapist often seems to have a magic touch.

Massage works on the soft tissues, muscles, and ligaments of the body. It stimulates circulation and the function of the nervous system and helps to lower blood pressure. It can soothe muscle tension and headaches and can help relieve insomnia. Massage is particularly beneficial after exercise. During a workout, waste products build up in the muscles. It can take the lymphatic system days to wash them away. Massage speeds up this process by improving the circulation of blood and lymph.

There are two main types of massage: shiatsu and Swedish. Shiatsu was developed in Japan at about the same time that acupuncture began to flourish in China. This massage involves finger pressure that stimulates the acupuncture points along the body's meridians. One form of shiatsu firmly massages certain areas of the body to stimulate the flow of energy and restore balance. Another form involves the use of a single fingertip to stimulate acupuncture points. The purpose of shiatsu is to alter the flow of energy within the body, and it works along the same principle as acupuncture. Shiatsu therapists also emphasize the importance of good nutrition and positive mental outlook, and they encourage clients to make lifestyle changes that promote greater health. Shiatsu can be combined with chiropractic to maximize its healing effects.

Swedish massage, which is more common in the West, involves four essential techniques, with the underlying premise that the hands should not lose contact with the body. Swedish massage is effective because of its continual, rhythmic motions. These are the basic techniques.

Effleurage: Rhythmic stroking with open hands, with movements directed toward the heart; this motion soothes and relaxes the body.

Percussion: Brisk rhythmic movements with alternate hands that include cupping, hacking (with sides of hands), pummeling (with fists), clapping, and plucking; this stimulates the skin and circulation.

Petrissage: Deep movement that involves lifting, rolling, squeezing, and pressing the skin; this stimulates muscles and fatty tissues, stretching taut muscles to relax them.

Pressure: As the thumbs, fingertips, or heel of the hand make small, pressured circular movements, friction stimulates superficial tissue.

When you visit a massage therapist, he or she probably will not take a detailed physical history, but you should inform him or her of any pains, illnesses, injuries, or recent surgeries you have had. The therapist usually will begin with the feet or back and will allow you a few moments to get used to the sensation of being touched and kneaded. It should be a thoroughly pleasurable treat!

Sessions are usually one hour long and cost approximately $30 to $70. Therapeutic massage is covered by some insurance companies when it is required by a doctor for the treatment of a particular ailment or injury due to an automobile or work-related accident. Massage is generally entirely safe, but you should not use it if the following conditions exist:

- Infectious, open wounds or bruises
- Varicose veins
- Fever
- Inflamed joints or acute arthritis
- Thrombosis or phlebitis (could disturb blood clot)

Massage and Pain

By itself, massage is not an appropriate treatment for chronic pain. It is, however, a soothing adjunct to all other natural therapies and cetainly can be part of your pain-management program.

Reflexology

Reflexology is a technique of deeply massaging the soles of the feet and hands in order to affect various parts of the body that are ailing. It was developed in China and India at the same time that acupuncture originated. Reflexology was brought to England in the twentieth century by Dr. William Fitzgerald, who called it zone therapy. In the United States Eunice Ingham developed Fitzgerald's teachings in the 1930s. Today, reflexology is growing in popularity, with schools located in Europe and the United States. Many practitioners of reflexology also perform chiropractic, osteopathy, and homeopathy.

Reflexology works on the premise that internal organs share the same nerve supplies as certain corresponding areas of the skin. Practitioners believe that the entire body is represented on the feet, primarily on the soles. By pressing the proper points on the feet, one can stimulate the organ associated with that point. These points are not the same as acupuncture points or meridians, many of which are not even represented on the feet.

During a reflexology session, the client will lie on a massage table while the practitioner feels the feet for granule-like substances deep within them. These "crystals" are actually waste deposits that build up in the nerve endings and capillaries and restrict the free flow of blood. The reflexology treatment breaks up the deposits so that they can be flushed from the body.

As the reflexologist "reads" the feet, he or she can determine which organs are affected. The patient will usually feel pain when a particular point is pressed, and sometimes in the corresponding organ or area of the body. The practitioner applies pressure with the edge of the thumb or finger and rotates it clockwise. The pressure is deep but should not be too painful. A session usually lasts from thirty to ninety minutes, and a client may require several sessions. Reflexology is beneficial for functional disorders that can be reversed, such as sinus problems, constipation, asthma, bladder problems, headaches, and stress.

PSYCHOTHERAPY

Psychotherapy, or "talk treatment," is an invaluable natural therapy for fostering and maintaining overall health. There has been much discussion about the mind/body connection. Although this has been an inherent part of holistic medicine throughout the world over time, orthodox Western medicine is realizing more and more the power of the mind and the importance of psychological treatments.

Mental health is important to physical health and vice versa. Emotional problems cause stress, which evokes physical symptoms and illness; physical illness, likewise, can cause a person to become depressed or lose energy and motivation. Doctors and patients are increasingly aware of the interplay of the mind and body and that in fact they may be inseparable, or one and the same.

Psychotherapy often requires you to talk about your feelings and problems, but it also can involve action, such as finding ways to alter your patterns of behavior. Treatment can be conducted on an individual basis between therapist and client, or it can be held within a group format. Group therapy allows clients to support and help each other, which can be just as valuable as receiving guidance from a therapist. People who seek out psychological treatment are not necessarily sick. They may simply be seeking greater understanding about themselves and their behavior.

There are many different kinds of psychotherapy, and some are more beneficial than others for treating particular disorders or problems. You may not hit upon the right therapy immediately, but don't give up. Success and progress in psychotherapy often take much time. If you really feel it's not working for you (and you've discussed this with the therapist), try a different therapist, and you might get better results. Psychotherapy, like many holistic, natural treatments, requires a willingness on the part of patients to be open to the treatment and to help themselves. You might go to a psychotherapist or counselor with the hope that the therapist will "cure" you. In fact, it takes work by both the therapist and the client in order for the treatment to be effective. The following sections list the major types of psychotherapy.

Supportive Psychotherapy

In this treatment, you can openly discuss your problems and feelings in a trusted, comfortable environment. The therapist should be a good listener who allows you the opportunity to vent your feelings, and who may make suggestions or point out insights that will give you a sense of support, without the feeling of being judged.

Exploratory Psychotherapy

This kind of treatment encourages you to explore your problems and issues, rather than just airing them. The therapist is usually active in the discussion and will let you know if you are avoiding a particular issue. Many healthy people pursue exploratory therapy as a way of learning more about themselves or to deal with a particular issue or aspect of their lives that they feel needs resolving or improvement.

Psychoanalysis

This treatment, which was originated by Sigmund Freud at the turn of the century, has taken a variety of forms. In classical psychoanalysis, you lie on a couch and talk freely about feelings, dreams, or whatever comes to mind. The psychoanalyst interprets what you say in terms of your childhood experiences and relationship with your parents. Psychoanalysis is usually intensive and long-term.

Other forms of psychoanalytic treatment focus on how your early emotional experiences have affected your current feelings and perceptions of yourself and relationships. This kind of therapy can help free you from pent-up or repressed childhood anger, frustration, hurt, and dependency. By working through these feelings, you will gain a greater sense of self-understanding and self-esteem.

Gestalt Therapy

Introduced in the United States by Fritz Perls in the 1950s, this "humanistic" therapy believes that the present moment, not the past, is most important, and that every person is responsible for his or her actions and has the ability to change them. In a session, if something from the past is bothersome, the therapist will help you bring it into the present. Gestalt therapists use many techniques to increase your awareness of yourself in the moment. For instance, if you are crying in a session, the therapist might ask you to speak to your tears. Merely talking about them promotes greater distancing between yourself and your emotions. Another Gestalt technique is for you to behave in a session opposite from the way you feel. For example, if you are very shy, the therapist might ask you to act like an outgoing person. Doing this will allow you to become aware of a part of yourself that exists but has remained undeveloped or repressed.

Behavioral Therapy

Behavioral therapists believe that all behavior is learned either through conditioning or the reinforcement of specific actions. For instance, if your mother taught you when you were growing up that all animals are dirty, you might develop a fear of animals, such as dogs. When the behavior you learned is negative or maladaptive, adverse psychological symptoms (in this example, a phobia) can result. Behavioral therapy can teach you new ways of behaving to help you live a more positive, happy, and productive life.

Behavioral therapy can resolve phobias, sexual dysfunction, inhibitions, and increase self-assertiveness. The therapist will help you learn new behaviors to replace those that are maladaptive. One method is called *operant conditioning*, by which new behaviors are rewarded and undesirable ones are ignored. In the *modeling* technique, the therapist "models," or displays for you to copy, the new behavior you are to practice. *Systemic desensitization* is a step-by-step process to help relieve specific fears or inhibitions.

Cognitive Therapy

This therapy was developed by American psychologist Aaron Beck in the 1960s. *Cognition* refers to a person's thinking, perception, and memory. If the therapist views your cognition as the cause of your emotional problems, the therapy will try to alter your perceptions and thoughts about yourself in order to alleviate the symptoms or problems. For example, if you were constantly denigrated by your father when you were growing up, chances are you developed a low self-esteem and often feel worthless. A cognitive therapist would point out evidence to the contrary, emphasizing your achievements that prove your self-worth.

Couples Therapy

Those who are married or involved in a serious intimate relationship know that even the best relationships require work. In couples therapy, you can visit a therapist either together or separately in order to understand and resolve tensions that exist within your relationship. Therapy can be useful to both heterosexual and homosexual couples.

Family Therapy

Families are intricate, dynamic networks that often require an objective outsider to help clear the air or resolve conflicts. When one or more family members has a problem, it often throws the entire unit into crisis, and this is when therapy can be beneficial. A family therapist is able to observe how the family operates together and can help the members understand not only how to deal with each other but their own roles within the family.

Just as it is important to find the right kind of therapy, it is equally important to build a good relationship with your therapist. As with other kinds of relationships, this can happen spontaneously, or it may take time. Within the emotional context of therapy, it is often difficult to discern how you feel about your therapist. Bear in mind that it is valid and important to discuss the feelings you have toward your therapist with him or her. This might provide insight as to how you relate to others.

The different kinds of therapists are distinguished by their training. *Psychotherapist* is a general term that refers to anyone who practices psychotherapy. A *psychiatrist* is a medical doctor who is trained in psychotherapy and can prescribe drugs for treating mental disorders. A *clinical psychologist* holds a doctoral degree in psychology and has training in psychotherapy. He or she cannot prescribe medicine, and may specialize in a particular type of therapy, such as psychoanalytic, behavioral, and so on. A *psychoanalyst* is a psychiatrist or psychologist who is specially trained in psychoanalysis.

You can seek psychotherapy from a private therapist or from a mental health center or clinic. Fees vary according to the practitioner, though some are willing to use a sliding scale—that is, they will charge a fee based on your income and the amount you are able to afford. Some insurance policies provide a psychotherapy benefit, while others do not. If your policy does, find out whether there is a limit to the number of sessions or if there is a cap on the amount of coverage provided each year.

Psychotherapy and Pain

The type of psychotherapy most beneficial to chronic pain patients depends on many factors. In various instances, all have been effective in the treatment of chronic pain syndromes. While exploratory psychoanalysis and Gestalt therapy have been found to be very effective in helping some chronic pain patients uncover hidden psychological causes of their pain, cognitive-behavioral therapy along with couples, family, and support therapies are used most commonly to help remedy these persistent conditions.

Cognitive-Behavioral Therapy and the Treatment of Pain

After your doctor visits, medications, and perhaps surgeries, what do you do when you still feel pain? Your personal response to this question is key to the use of cognitive-behavioral therapy. Ask yourself now:

1. Have you had to adjust your activities and lifestyle as a result of your pain?
2. Do you think about your pain almost every day?
3. Have you relinquished to others small tasks, such as answering the phone?
4. Is bed rest one of your primary pain-management techniques?
5. Do you talk about your pain?
6. Do you tell yourself or others that your pain is the worst thing that has ever happened to you?

If you answer "yes" to just one of these questions, you probably are not a candidate for pain management through cognitive-behavioral therapy, but if you see yourself in several of these situations, you may find help through this kind of therapy. Cognitive-behavioral therapy focuses on negative and/or noncoping thoughts and actions caused by persistent pain and repeated treatment failures and the tendency of pain sufferers to focus their attention on their pain so intently that it comes to dominate their lives to the exclusion of other activities.

When obsession with pain allows it to become the controlling life force, a great sense of helplessness and hopelessness can result. Researchers have long noted the connection between these feelings and the high rate of depression. But contrary to what you may believe, problems such as depression and disability generally do not resolve on their own when treatment focuses solely on reducing pain. Comprehensive management of chronic pain syndromes requires first a recognition of pain as a complex perception and then an appreciation of the significant role of thoughts and behavior in the development, maintenance, and alleviation of chronic pain.

In cognitive-behavioral therapy, you are encouraged to identify through self-monitoring your negative thoughts and behaviors, challenge them, and replace them with more appropriate pain-management strategies. Once this is done, you're better able to accept alternative pain-relief remedies, change your lifestyle of inactivity and declining strength, improve your relationships, look for meaningful work, and increase your overall wellness. All of this can be accomplished without focusing directly on the pain itself.

The cognitive-behavioral management of chronic pain is most appropriate for treating chronic benign pain if you are currently medically stable and are not a candidate for further aggressive medical treatment. The treatment focuses on the mental and physical reactions to pain and contains few features that are specific to any particular type of pain. Therefore, therapy can be effective regardless of the location, duration, frequency, or intensity of your pain.

Treatment may be provided on an inpatient or outpatient basis. Inpatient settings, however, are often recommended because they provide the opportunity for greater structure and control over the program, and the clinicians work together to coordinate all aspects of the program. For most patients, a combination of a brief hospitalization followed by an intensive short-term outpatient program is best.

Repeatedly, research and clinical studies have found that cognitive-behavioral therapy offers many benefits to chronic pain patients. A 1985 study by Moore and Chaney highlights the success of this approach. Their results demonstrate that cognitive-behavioral treatment is successful not only in reducing the number of times a person complains about his or her pain, but also in reducing use of the health-care system; in reducing pain behaviors such as moaning, sleeping, complaining, and limping that are observed by spouses; and in improving physical functioning, body control, and movement.

In practice, cognitive therapy and behavioral therapy

frequently are used together. In your therapy sessions you will most likely learn pain-management strategies using this dual approach. For your own information, however, consider how each kind of therapy explained in the next sections works to relieve pain.

Beck's Cognitive Therapy

"Cognition" is a word used to refer to a person's thinking, perception, and memory. For the pain patient, the basis of cognitive therapy (developed by American psychologist Aaron Beck in the late 1960s) is this: People who think they can control their pain, who avoid thinking the worst about their condition, and who believe they are not severely disabled appear to function better than those who do not. Cognitive therapy can be extremely effective in treating the emotional distress that results from the effects of chronic pain.

To begin therapy, you might be asked to keep track of how you think about your pain. The following chart will give you an idea of the kind of cognitive distortions that support pain.

Cognitive Distortion	Example
Do you catastrophize?	"This is the worst pain in the world." "My life is ruined." "I'll never be myself again."
Do you overgeneralize?	"No one understands me." "This will never end."

Do you personalize?	"Leave it to me to have this kind of pain."
	"I guess I deserve to live like this."
Do you obsess?	"This is awful. This is terrible. I can't stand this."
Do you give power of cure to God or wishful thinking?	"God, please make this pain stop."
	"I wish I didn't have this pain."

All of these self-talk statements actually can increase the perception of physical pain. They even can bring on pain that's not being felt yet just by anticipating it. Research conducted by Dr. Dennis Turk at the Center for Pain Evaluation and Treatment at the University of Pittsburgh School of Medicine found that this anticipatory distress— the things you say and think about your pain when you're not feeling it yet—can produce muscle tension that may actually bring on pain. That's why if you worry that your pain will keep you awake tonight, it surely will. If you fret that your pain will be incapacitating on the day of an important event, it will. As a person living with chronic pain, it's vital to your pain management that you understand the clear relationship between the way you think about your pain and the way you feel it.

Cognitive therapy will help you to recognize your own self-talk attitudes and identify the negative statements you say to yourself. Some attitudes are subconscious and more difficult to identify, but your therapist will encourage you to start focusing on what you say to yourself. Then you'll learn to challenge the negative statements with positive, realistic ones. For example:

Imagine you are preparing for a holiday gathering of family and friends in your home. As you rush to get everything ready, you begin to feel your back pain. Now self-talk begins:

"Oh, no. Now this lovely holiday is going to be ruined because of this pain. I won't be able to enjoy the company of my family and friends. I may even have to spend the day alone in my bed, while everyone else celebrates without me. I prepared all this food and went to all this trouble, and will be left alone to suffer. I'm just not meant to enjoy the good things in life. This always happens to me."

Cognitive therapy will teach you to redirect this dialogue by recognizing the negative thoughts and challenging them with positive, constructive self-statements. You might change the above dialogue like this:

"Oh, no, my back pain is starting up again. Well, I won't let it ruin my holiday. I have my family and friends around me today and their love and support will help me get through this. Today is one day I won't go lie in my bed. There's no reason for me to miss this celebration. I worked hard to prepare this food and I'm going to enjoy it. I deserve to have a wonderful day."

When you combine this kind of positive self-talk with a few relaxation strategies (see pages 91–107), you will find yourself in control of your pain and your life.

Another cognitive strategy is called distraction. Although very simple in execution, this strategy is a commonly overlooked pain-relief technique. It seems that our mind can hold only one topic in consciousness at a time. You can choose consciously to attend to your pain by thinking about it, *or* you can choose consciously to think of something else. When you feel your pain taking up an undue degree of your mental attention, distract your mind away from the pain by going for a walk, talking to a friend, watching TV, or playing cards. Anything that requires your mental and physical attention can be used as a cognitive distraction strategy.

Historically the cognitive aspect of pain has received little attention from the pain-care physician. This is unfortunate because many experts believe that pain is a private, subjective experience. Therefore, a report of pain is the end result of a cognitive process. To deal with your pain, you can alter the way you think about your pain. Cognitive therapy can help you do this.

Behavioral Therapy

Behavioral therapists maintain that all behavior is learned and that certain learned behaviors promote and aggravate pain. Currently behavioral intervention is widely regarded as important, if not essential, in the treatment of patients with chronic benign pain. Fortunately, therapists can help you identify the things you do that keep you stuck in the cycle of pain and teach you new behaviors to replace those that support your pain.

When a given behavior causes a positive thing to happen, naturally you will want to repeat it to gain that positive feedback again. Each time the behavior elicits the desired response, it's reinforced, and this encourages you to repeat it again with greater intensity, frequency, or both. On the other hand, if an unpleasant thing follows a particular action, you are quite likely to avoid performing that action. Sounds logical, doesn't it?

This model is particularly applicable to chronic pain behavior. It's clear that as pain behavior becomes positively reinforced over time, it becomes the desired, natural behavior.

Behavior modification is designed to break the unwholesome behavior patterns of chronic pain patients that have previously been rewarded: drug taking, avoidance of activity, dependence on others, and preoccupation with pain. Behavioral therapy encourages and rewards the very opposite of these behaviors: responsibility instead of irresponsibility, independence instead of dependence, activity instead of lethargy, and the desire to free oneself from pain and not be bound to it.

The immediate goals of behavioral therapy are directly pain related. You will identify your personal pain behaviors:

- Do you avoid physical activity to "protect" your pain?

- Have you stopped socializing because of your pain?

- Do you want others to take care of you?

- Do you rely on medication for pain relief?

- Do you often groan, limp, rub, brace yourself, or talk about your pain?

- Do you get attention by talking about your pain?

- Do you use your pain to avoid undesirable activities?

- Do you sustain your pain in the hope of gaining monetary compensation?

These are all pain behaviors that you've adopted as a way to manage your pain. Some of them are conscious behaviors, some unconscious. Either way, they change the way you live your life.

After you identify the pain behaviors you've developed, behavioral therapy will help you cope with your pain in ways that will undo your learned pain behaviors. For example, consider a pain patient with arthritis who has learned to cope with pain by lying in bed and taking pain medication whenever the pain became intense. In a typical program, this patient would be given specific daily assignments, such as exercise, walking, or household chores.

These tasks would be ones the patient is capable of doing and ideally enjoys. The frequency, duration, and intensity of activities is explicitly explained ahead of time, and it is understood that the activities must be carried out as agreed before the patient can take pain medication. In this way, the pain-relief "reward" is contingent on the performance of the necessary activities. As the treatment continues, the patient is required to become progressively more active until a desired level of activity is reached.

Behavior modification rewards you with praise, attention, and support for positive changes. It withholds these things when you utilize negative pain behaviors. This is the core of the behavior modification technique.

Cognitive and behavioral therapies are combined in comprehensive programs because the chronic pain patient's beliefs regarding capabilities are strongly related to coping efforts. If you *think* you can exercise for twenty minutes, you will give it a good try. But if you *think,* "I can't do that; I'll be in too much pain," your efforts will be minimal and unsuccessful. Many studies have shown that pain patients' beliefs about their ability to perform various acts may better predict what they actually do than beliefs about how effective these behaviors will be in reducing pain. This seems to indicate that the time you spend talking about and thinking about the benefits of exercise, for example, might be better spent *doing* exercise, because seeing is believing.

About 65 percent of chronic sufferers who receive cognitive-behavioral therapy show significant improvement. This includes helpless patients who were previously crippled by chronic pain, with past histories involving unsuccessful surgeries for pain and multiple-drug misuse. If these programs have been carried through to a successful conclusion, they result in patients feeling less physical pain and more physically fit. They increase well-being, self-esteem, and personal happiness.

Along with cognitive-behavioral therapies, there are other kinds of psychotherapy that can be very beneficial to the chronic pain patient.

Supportive Psychotherapy

Once you've decided to change your life and adopt an active, self-controlled approach to coping with chronic pain, you might benefit greatly from a supportive environment. In supportive therapy, a client is able to discuss problems and feelings in trusted, comfortable surroundings. The therapist is a good listener who allows the client to vent and may make suggestions or point out insights that give the client a sense of support, without the feeling of being judged.

You also might consider joining a support group at a local hospital or pain clinic. People in pain often feel socially isolated and misunderstood, and support groups offer ways to confront these feelings and gain social support. Meeting with others who share fears and experiences can be quite therapeutic. A support group gives pain sufferers a place to learn how others cope; it also offers a sounding board for venting anger and frustration, and it gives an audience for the pain stories that few people outside the group want to listen to over and over again. A support group helps to validate a person's perception of something that's really indescribable, and it offers a place to learn more about how others manage and live with their pain.

Support groups come in all shapes and sizes. They may be structured and medically supervised; they may be informal social gatherings; they may be educational or cathartic.

But in the end they are a gathering of sympathetic people who offer each other support. If you're interested in joining a support group, ask your doctor or therapist to help you find one in your area.

Family and/or Couples Therapy

Your chronic pain does not affect only you. It affects everyone in your family, and therefore it is most helpful if everyone has an opportunity to gain insight into the intricate dynamic network of dependency that you may have established. In many cases the spouse or partner and other family members are co-conspirators in the development and maintenance of your pain behaviors. These behaviors (that will prolong the pain experience) are encouraged when family members take over responsibilities, allow avoidance behaviors to continue, and offer the reward of sympathy and attention for verbal expressions of pain. Nagging, threatening, or coercing actually can reinforce pain and disability because, after all, even this kind of attention is still attention.

A family or couples therapist is able to observe how the family operates together. He or she can help the members understand not only how to deal with each other but their own roles within the family. Thus, the family dynamics related to the reinforcement of your pain can be uncovered by the therapist and corrected so that family members do not unwittingly reinforce behaviors or beliefs that enhance your pain. And together, you can all work in ways that will help you overcome your negative pain habits.

RELAXATION THERAPY

Relaxation therapy doesn't mean bed rest. This mode of natural medicine involves various self-help techniques that actually can control the involuntary workings of the nervous system that are known to support and aggravate pain. These techniques can help you manage your pain by influencing blood pressure, heart rate, respiration, and metabolism—all seemingly involuntary physiological functions that power the chronic pain cycle.

In addition to their effect on these bodily functions, relaxation techniques can break the stress/pain cycle by decreasing muscle tension, improving your sense of pain control, relieving anxiety, encouraging restful sleep, and in some cases stimulating the body to release its own natural painkillers, endorphins.

The roots of the body's physical response to stress go back to our primitive days. In the era of cave people, the difference between bringing an animal home to eat and being eaten by the animal was a person's ability to react quickly to danger. The human body had to be able to prepare for fight or flight at a moment's notice. To do this, breathing became faster and shallower to bring more oxygen into the human body quickly. The heartbeat increased to push that oxygen and increased blood sugar through the bloodstream rapidly. And the blood flow was redirected from the internal organs and surface of the body to the deep muscles, which needed more energy to prepare for the emergency.

Those people who had quick stress-response systems survived. The problem is that this stress response, which was designed to promote the physical activity of running away or fighting, is no longer appropriate for us. Today, we no longer need extra oxygen directed to our deep muscles when we feel stress or pain, yet it still happens. Our body prepares us to fight, but most often we have no visible foe. So what happens? Our heart beats rapidly; our blood pressure becomes elevated; our muscles tighten; and after a while our body begins to wear down. We develop physical illnesses such as ulcers, headaches, heart palpitations, backaches, rashes, colitis, allergies, asthma, heart disease, diabetes, chronic pain syndromes, and (as found in the latest research) even cancer.

Research fully supports what you already know: Chronic pain can be extremely stressful. But to use relaxation therapy successfully, you must first acknowledge that stress contributes to the intensity, frequency, and duration of your pain, and then recognize that it is a treatable condition you can control. This is important because it has been proven that people who feel they have no control over their pain feel the highest degree of stress and therefore pain. If you want to use relaxation therapy in your pain-management program, you can no longer sidestep responsibility by saying such things as "I can't help getting so tense" or "I've always been the kind of person who gets stressed out." Of course, no one can completely eliminate the stress of daily living or the stress of pain, but you can learn to manage it. This and the following chapters give you several proven ways you *can* control the way you react to stress.

How does reducing stress reduce pain? Well, it happens in several ways:

1. Self-regulated stress management improves your sense of control over your pain. Cognitive therapists assure us that the way we think about our pain affects the way we feel it. Relaxation techniques put you in charge; they give you an active role in managing your pain. This alone reduces the feelings of helplessness and hopelessness that support and maintain pain.

2. Relaxation techniques reduce anxiety. It's difficult to think positively and continue your pain-management regimen each day if you are chronically anxious and tense. Relaxation techniques give you a sense of ease and determination.

3. Relaxation therapy enhances sleep. Chronic pain is the great robber of sleep; relaxation techniques calm the body, improve circulation, lower anxiety levels, and promote peaceful rest.

4. Relaxation reduces the sensation of pain by decreasing muscle tension. Studies have shown that stress-related muscle tension often is greatest at the body's most vulnerable site—the source of chronic pain.

5. Relaxation therapy improves overall well-being. If a stress response is chronic, the constant presence of adrenaline pumping into your system begins to wear down the body's immunological system. You need a strong and healthy body to manage chronic pain. Relaxation techniques can help you achieve that physiological state.

Most relaxation techniques can be practiced anywhere at your convenience without special apparati or devices. But to learn the strategies, practice them in a comfortable, quiet spot, free of distractions. Then you can practice some anytime and anywhere. Some are portable and can be used when you find yourself in the middle of a stressful situation. They are always handy and can be pulled out when you feel your pain level begin to increase. They are yours to use not only in times of emergency but to maintain a healthy and calm state of being.

You'll need to experiment a bit to find out which relaxation techniques work best for you. Some take effort and practice, so don't give up too soon on any one. Try them all;

give them a chance to prove their worth. Then choose a few that you feel comfortable doing. Relaxation therapy is a lifelong skill that will improve the quality of your life, not only in relation to pain management but in all areas of health and well-being.

Guided Visual Imagery

Because we all daydream and nightdream, we already know we have an internal world that we can experience in both positive and negative ways. Guided imagery requires you to go to that inner world and construct a place where you'll feel safe and relaxed whenever you imagine yourself being there.

To better understand how guided imagery works in a positive way, let's first take a look at how a negative image can produce its own stress. Imagine this:

It is 2:00 A.M. You've just woken in great pain for the second time that night. You've been very cranky this week because you've been lying awake in pain for the last five nights and your doctor says there's nothing more he can do. You're especially bothered by your pain now because in the morning you want to look and feel alert for a special and important meeting. Just as you lay your head back down on the pillow determined to sleep, the pain intensifies and you moan out load. Your spouse rolls away, annoyed. You feel a growing surge of rage; your heart is pounding, and you begin to cry. Your only thought is "I just can't stand another minute of this!"

If you close your eyes and imagine all this happening to you, you'll cause an increase in your stress level just by thinking about it. The internal experience alone—just the image—can produce a stress response.

Since a negative image can produce stress so easily, it's

only logical that a positive image can reduce it. The core belief of the guided imagery approach to stress reduction is that imagining a positive experience can stop, interrupt, or prevent a physical stress reaction.

To do this, create a positive image in your mind that represents a safe and relaxing environment. Practice visiting it over and over again. Then when you're stressed, you can go there just briefly and benefit from the relaxed feeling it gives you. For example, you may find this image soothing:

> *I am stretched out on the ocean beach. The sun is warm on my body. When it gets too strong, I have an umbrella for protection. I feel the warmth of the sand on my fingertips. I see the calm ocean touching the shore. I can smell the salt of the ocean, and I can taste the sea air. On my beach there's just the right number of people —I'm not crowded or lonely. On my beach there are no sand crabs or flies. I feel just wonderful. It's an ideal place that I can visit with all my senses anytime I want. Even when I'm in the middle of a crowd with my eyes wide open, I can go to my beach.*

This safe place happens to be a beach—yours can be anywhere. It can be in your family room by the fireplace, the woods by a stream, the park down the street. It can be anywhere, but keep this in mind:

- Make the place real. When you're stressed or in pain, you won't be able to relate to an alien planet.
- Involve all of your senses. Make sure all the smells and the things you touch, taste, hear, and see in this environment are pleasing to you.
- Go to this place often. The more you practice increasing the quality of your image, the more you can

rely on it when you're in pain. It will become a
practiced response.

Another kind of guided imagery is used to battle chronic
pain under the guidance of a trained therapist. Introduced
in the 1970s to help athletes and musicians perform better,
the method has won increasing acceptance among some
doctors as a way to manage chronic pain. Patients are
taught how their immune system is affected by their disease, pain, and stress. Then with cues from the therapist or
a tape recording, they learn mentally to visualize their condition and "see" the body fighting against the pain and
restoring comfort and health. A person suffering from the
pain of arthritis in the hands, for example, might mentally
see her inflamed and stiff joints regain flexible, fluid movement without deformity or pain. This mental picture temporarily can convince the brain that there is no need to
transmit pain messages.

Autogenic Training

Autogenic training is based on self-generated statements
that help you redirect your focus of concentration until you
have blocked out the external stress trigger, which in your
case is the sensation of pain.

Give this example a try: In your mind's eye focus on a
part of your body that is not in pain—let's say your right
arm and right hand. Try to experience them completely by
taking a journey through them. Feel how they touch the
chair. Feel your arm hair touch the upholstery, your ring
touch your finger, your shirt lie on your shoulder. When
you are completely aware of your arm and hand, repeat a
relaxing phrase over and over again. Try something like:

My arm is heavy and warm. The warmth is flowing into my hand. Or *My right arm is light and cool. It feels like it's floating.* (Or whatever statement describes how you feel when you are relaxed.)

Then stop and take a look at your hand and arm, and describe to yourself how they feel. Do they feel warm and heavy? Light? What does the sensation of relaxation feel like? Tell yourself:

My heartbeat is calm and regular. My breathing is relaxed and comfortable.

This process will take your mind away from your pain and place all your powers of concentration on something else. The passive repetition of these phrases coupled with the mental visualization of the desired goal can lead to a 10 percent drop in pulse and blood pressure and an increase of one to two degrees in skin temperature of hands and feet, better blood flow in abdominal organs, slowed breathing, decreased metabolic rate, slowed brain-wave activity, and a sense of well-being.

Deep Breathing

Because the body needs oxygen to fuel its stress response, you can reduce or short circuit the stress you feel by regaining control of your breathing. Athletes often do this just before a race begins or as they are about to get up to bat.

Follow these instructions to stop the rapid breathing that accompanies a stress response.

- Put your hand on your stomach.
- Take a deep breath from the bottom of your stomach.

- Feel it fill you with warm air.
- Feel your hand rise with your stomach muscles.
- Breathe in as you silently count to five.
- Let the air go. Don't push it out. Let it go gently to the count of five.
- When you let out the air, smile.
- Do this sequence two times in a row.
- Then breathe regularly (rhythmically and comfortably).
- Breathe deeply again after you have let a minute or two go by.
- Repeat this deep-breathing/regular-breathing cycle two or three times, or as often as needed, until you find your breathing has returned to a natural and comfortable pace.

It's recommended that you smile when you exhale because smiling is a natural mood elevator. While you're smiling, it's difficult to be stressed. Try this experiment: Think nasty thoughts while you're smiling. Don't just say nasty words, but actually think and feel nasty thoughts while you're smiling. Isn't it hard? That's why you can help your body ease its tension if you smile when you exhale.

Deep breathing is a strategy you can use anywhere. No one around needs to know you're practicing a stress-reduction technique. It's a technique you can engage in whenever you feel your pain increasing and your body tensing. Without changing your thoughts or actions, deep breathing will change your body's reaction to pain.

Meditation

Meditation can be used to enhance the effectiveness of deep breathing. Deep breathing can arrest a pain-stress response, but too often the effort is sabotaged by the appearance of negative or stressful thoughts. If your mind continues to concentrate on your pain or stress while you breathe deeply, you are unlikely to reach your goal of total relaxation. To counter this intrusion of stressful thoughts, add meditation to your deep-breathing exercises. There are many established programs of meditation, but for a sample of a basic meditative style follow these instructions.

Choose a word or phrase (known as your mantra) that you will focus on during your meditation. This may be the word "one" or "fun" or anything you choose. Then as you expel your deep breath, say this word silently to yourself. As you breathe in, your mind may still have a stressful thought, but as you breathe out, switch your attention back to your mantra. With practice, you'll be able to breathe and meditate without stressful thoughts bothering you. This stress-free, relaxed time will give your body opportunity to rejuvenate and calm itself so that you can uphold your commitment to your pain-management regimen.

Progressive Muscle Relaxation

In stressful situations many people describe the way they feel as being "tied up in knots." Because of the way our muscles react to stress, this actually is true. Progressive muscle relaxation will help you untie the knots by teaching you how to recognize muscle tension and then how to relax the involved muscles. Then, when you feel stress in physical pain, you can relax those muscles that are aggravating your pain. By practicing progressive muscle relaxation, you will learn what it feels like when stress begins to manifest itself in muscle tension. Then when your muscles do begin to tense involuntarily, you will be able to identify the problem area and stop the stress attack.

To begin, tense and relax the various muscle groups listed in the table. Maintain that tension for five to ten seconds so you have time to feel how whole parts of your body are involved in tension. When you have a muscle group tensed, let your mind's eye experience that part of your body. If you're tensing your arm, for example, press your forearm down against the table. Feel where the tension goes out through your fingertips, up onto your shoulders, right into your neck—then relax. Feel the experience of letting go—of consciously relaxing your muscles.

There is no magic in this list of muscle groups. Pick ones that make sense for your needs and practice until you're well acquainted with the feeling of tension in each one. Then give the method a chance to relieve the stress you feel in your life and the pain it causes.

The next time you're lying in bed at 2:00 in the morning listening to your pain, let your mind's eye go through your body to ascertain the location of the tension. For many people it's commonly in the lower back, neck, or shoulders; for others it's in and around the forehead or the jaw area. When you've found your tense area, use the skill of progressive muscle relaxation to ease the muscles that have become a pain trigger for you.

Repeat the following exercises three times with the listed muscle groups.

Muscle Group	Exercise
right hand	Make a fist.
right forearm	Press down.
left hand	Make a fist.
left forearm	Press down.

shoulders	Shrug.
neck	Lean your head back and roll it from side to side.
head:	
jaw	Bite down lightly.
tongue	Press on the roof of your mouth.
eyes	Squint.
forehead	Frown and raise your brows.
abdomen	Tighten your stomach as if someone were going to hit you.
back	Arch slightly.
right leg	Press down on the floor.
left leg	Press down on the floor.
toes	Curl under.

People with hypertension should not relax large groups of muscles. Doing so forces volumes of blood to return to the heart and increases blood pressure. Autogenic training is preferred for these individuals.

If you have medical complications, consult your physician or see a professional stress-management specialist for guidance.

Music

Not only can music soothe the savage beast, it can ease the suffering caused by chronic pain. Indeed, this readily available, low-cost/low-risk strategy has been identified as a form of auditory stimulation that can be effective in controlling pain. A 1981 study reported in the *Journal of Advanced Nursing* concluded that music decreases musculoskeletal, verbal, and physiological-autonomic pain reactions among postoperative patients during the first forty-eight hours. The studied group also used less pain-relief medications, indicating that music can be used to relieve or alleviate pain.

Auditory stimulation has a pronounced physiological effect on the body in at least two ways. It's possible that music may be related to the gate control theory of pain. Intense stimuli such as music can cause the production of endorphins that inhibit the release of neurotransmitters; this would stimulate the closure of the gate that allows pain messengers passage.

Music also can be used as a tactic of diversion. Diverting attention away from the pain decreases the body's adverse physiological responses to stress and tension. When this relaxation occurs, painful muscle tensing at the vulnerable site is decreased and the pain lessened.

Studies reporting the effectiveness of music as a treatment for chronic pain suggest a few simple guidelines for effectively using music therapy:

• Schedule a specific time for listening to music. Deciding to "listen to more music" is too general and unstructured to be of any benefit.

• Find a place where you can lie down or comfortably sit.

• If possible, use headphones to drown out environmental distractions.

- Choose any music at any volume that you find relaxing. Studies have found no difference in results from hard rock to "easy listening" music.
- Listen with positive expectations. If you believe music can ease your pain, it is more likely that it will.

Music as therapy can be an effective pain-relief remedy, but only as an adjunct to other natural remedies. It cannot, by itself, completely manage pain.

Laughter

In his book *Anatomy of an Illness as Perceived by the Patient*, Norman Cousins wrote, "Ten minutes of genuine belly laughter had an anesthetic effect that would give me at least two hours of pain-free sleep."

The reasons for this seemingly "miraculous" pain relief are probably a combination of several factors. Sustained laughter may very well stimulate the release of the body's natural painkillers, endorphins. It's also believed that the nervous system can hold only one kind of sensation at a time; it cannot simultaneously react to pleasure and tension. Therefore, laughter can transmit a positive and joyful message that overrides those of anxiety, stress, depression, and pain. At the same time, laughter provides a source of distraction that keeps the body's focus away from pain, relaxes the muscles that aggravate pain, and offers temporary but welcome pain relief.

Look for ways to include laughter in your day: Next time you're browsing through the video store, choose a comedy. If you have the choice of watching a TV crime story or a sitcom, choose the sitcom. Cultivate your sense of humor and laugh often. Pain is not funny, but laughter is its enemy.

HYPNOSIS

Moving from side-show entertainment to medical therapy has been a long journey for the art of hypnosis. First introduced by Austrian physician Franz Mesmer in the late eighteenth century, hypnosis was used to "mesmerize" patients with neuroses; throughout the nineteenth century it received much attention for its use in providing anesthesia during surgery. However, eventually the medical and psychological communities characterized it as nothing but heated imagination, and the therapy fell into disrepute for the remainder of the century. But indeed, today it has arrived into the mainstream of medical practice.

The American Society of Clinical Hypnosis says that there are now an estimated 15,000 to 20,000 practitioners among all types of medical specialists, including family practitioners, anesthesiologists, orthopedists, surgeons, psychologists, and psychiatrists. While all agree that by itself hypnosis has limited curative powers, hypnosis has proven itself very effective in treating a wide variety of physical and mental ailments.

Exactly how hypnosis works is unclear. Practitioners guide patients into a hypnotic state by having them focus on a particular mental image, a soothing voice, or an object. Once in a trance, thought patterns are temporarily suspended. One theory suggests that the limbic system—the brain region related to emotional responses—is stimulated under hypnosis, rendering the patient very receptive to the hypnotist's suggestions.

Perception can be altered in varied ways under the trance of hypnosis. Individuals can become dissociated with respect to time; they can be led to make "involuntary" movements. They may experience imaginary phenomena or become dissociated from external reality. Some individuals experience amnesia or find they can recall the details of forgotten events. A few of these responses have been found to be particularly effective in helping people manage chronic pain.

The most common hypnotic approach to pain relief is through hypnotic dissociation. Although the body and mind ordinarily work as a whole and in harmony, dissociation can be used to control pain by separating the area of pain from the rest of the body. For example, a person may be hypnotized and led to believe that his painful arm feels quite numb, having no feeling at all. In this circumstance, sensation in the arm has become dissociated from the rest of the body. In the same way, if the joints of a woman's hand suffer the pain of arthritis, under hypnosis she can hold herself apart from the hand and become convinced that the painful hand really does not belong to her; it has "nothing to do with her" and causes her no pain.

Experts in the field believe hypnosis can be used as a pain-management strategy is several ways. It can change the perception of pain by:

- blocking awareness of pain by altering its perception
- substituting another feeling for a painful one
- displacing the pain sensation to a smaller, less vulnerable area of the body
- altering the meaning of pain so it is viewed as less debilitating and less important
- distorting time to control pain by helping patients perceive painful times as passing quickly
- suggesting amnesia so patients can forget periods of pain

Hypnosis does not work for everyone. The likelihood of being able to be hypnotized varies from one person to the next. Approximately 10 percent of the population is very hypnotizable and about half is relatively hypnotizable. A therapist may choose to administer a "test" of suggestibility before attempting to ease your pain with hypnosis, by giving a number of trial suggestions and observing how well you respond. He or she may choose to use a psychometric scale that measures various aspects of hypnotic phenomena such as dissociation, involuntary movement, amnesia, and suspension of judgment. Or the practitioner may decide to use the Hypnotic Induction Profile (HIP), created by Dr. Herbert Spiegel of Columbia University. This test uses the fairly simple eye-roll technique; it's believed that the higher you can roll your eyes upward while keeping the eyelids open, the more susceptible to hypnosis you will be. Also, suggestibility can be measured with Dr. Theodore's Creative Imagination Scale, which takes about eighteen minutes to administer.

If you find that you are open to the power of hypnosis, you might want to try this method as a pain-control strategy. Hypnosis is particularly effective in easing pain that is exacerbated by stress, tension, or anxiety or if the pain is psychogenic in origin. Through hypnosis, deep states of relaxation can be attained. This allows tense muscles to relax and blood circulation to flow smoothly, thus easing the pain of tension-based problems.

Hypnosis is renowned for its use in treating pain of psychogenic origin. It is well known that psychological stress can present itself as physical pain. Through hypnosis, patients can identify the psychological source of distress and thereby relieve or even eliminate the physical pain.

If you decide to use hypnosis as a part of your pain-management regimen, be sure to take some time to find a legitimate hypnotist. As of December 31, 1993, the American Society of Clinical Hypnosis has been certifying individuals in hypnosis. But because this program is so new, at this time most practitioners are not specially certified. But you can still avoid quackery by making sure your practitioner has some kind of professional degree. Whether the field of specialty is psychology, psychiatry, social work, specialty nursing, dentistry, or medicine, look for evidence of professional health-care training.

If you try hypnosis and are a good subject, you can expect the pain relief to last for several days after the session. If hypnosis is working, you'll find that, over time, the effects will last longer and longer. But because hypnosis is not a one-shot cure, it is expensive and inconvenient to rely continually on a practitioner for pain relief. Fortunately, you can learn the skill of hypnosis from your practitioner (or from any number of books on the subject) and eventually learn the art of self-hypnosis, which you can use whenever you're in need of pain relief.

BIOFEEDBACK

Biofeedback probably presents the greatest evidence of the mind's influence over the body. In a healthy person, physiological functions are performed and regulated by the brain and central nervous system. The mind, however, often interferes, such as under conditions of stress that produce tension in the body. Biofeedback can teach the patient to intervene under these conditions in order to restore balanced functioning in the body.

Conscious control can affect many body functions that can be measured accurately and continuously, such as heart rate, skin temperature, blood pressure, muscle tension, and brain waves. The biofeedback equipment that measures these functions includes the electroencephalograph (EEG), which records nerve and brain waves, the electromyograph (EMG), which registers muscle tension, and the galvanic skin resistance instrument (GSR), which detects the electrical conductivity of the skin to record states of arousal, excitement, or nervousness.

When you are hooked up to these machines, they convey information to you through signals that can be recognized and interpreted easily. For instance, when the instrument detects muscle tension, a red light might go on or a certain sound might be emitted to signal what is happening to you internally. You then can use this information, in addition to certain relaxation and imagery techniques, to begin controlling the muscle tension. The techniques that are used in combination with the biofeedback equipment include relaxation and autosuggestion exercises, visual imagery, and meditation. For example, if the equipment signals that your heart rate is increasing, you can use imagery, by imagining a calm, peaceful place, or meditate through the repeating of a mantra in order to relax your mind and body. In biofeedback treatment, therefore, the patient is not the object of the therapy, he or she *becomes* the therapy itself.

There are many applications for biofeedback, including stress-related illness, neuromuscular problems, and personal growth and increased self-awareness. Biofeedback can be effective treatment for emotional or behavioral problems, such as anxiety, depression, phobias, insomnia, tension headaches, and bruxism (teeth-grinding). It also can be used to treat illnesses considered by some professionals to be psychosomatic such as asthma, ulcers, colitis, diarrhea, cardiac arrhythmia, hypertension, Raynaud's syndrome, and migraines. Biofeedback can help victims of stroke, cerebral palsy, and muscle spasms in some functions of the muscles and movement. Since biofeedback increases your recognition and understanding of your total mind-body functioning, it also can be beneficial in enhancing personal growth and self-awareness.

Many general and psychiatric hospitals have biofeedback

clinics, and it is probably best to undergo treatments administered by a psychologist who is trained in biofeedback. A psychologist would be helpful in the process of developing greater self-awareness, and you might even consider combining biofeedback with psychotherapy.

When you begin biofeedback sessions, you should be informed about the equipment being used and the learning process and receive information about the muscles and the physiological functions involved in the treatment. Having this knowledge will help you to relax during the treatment and will probably enhance its success. Remember that while you must be an active participant in biofeedback, too much effort can produce unwanted stress. The key is to relax, using meditation, imagery, and other techniques, in order to focus fully on your internal states.

Biofeedback training can last weeks, months, or years, depending on your problem. Most people need at least six weeks' worth of sessions, which last from thirty to sixty minutes and can occur once a week or daily, again, depending on the need. The cost of biofeedback varies depending on your location, with an average cost of $75.00 per session. Check your insurance plan for coverage. You must learn to transfer what you learn from the biofeedback sessions to your daily life. It will take practice to begin to recognize the signs of trouble—such as muscle tension, headaches, and so on—and the situations in which they occur, and then to use the techniques that can relieve them without the biofeedback instrument. You probably will need periodic checkups in order to maintain the progress you have made.

Biofeedback for Chronic Pain

In cases of chronic pain, biofeedback has proven to be quite effective. In fact, it is arguably the most effective natural medicine remedy for chronic pain that is aggravated by stress and depression. As you are certainly aware, chronic pain can cause a person to feel a strong sense of helplessness and loss of control; biofeedback concretely demonstrates the extent to which a person can indeed control his or her body and thus pain. This forces the chronic pain sufferer to accept the underlying principle that governs all of natural medicine: There is an undeniable interrelationship between the body and mind. For many this realization is a harbinger of hope and is a stronger antidepressant than any prescribed medication.

Biofeedback has become one of the more widely used natural medicine remedies for chronic pain for several reasons. First, biofeedback allows you to take an active role in your treatment, unlike other, passive remedies such as acupuncture, massage, and reflexology. Active involvement in pain reduction has been found in and of itself to reduce the perception and tolerance of pain. The passive role that says "Someone else, please relieve my pain" promotes feelings of helplessness that fuel depression. Active involvement can empower you and give you a sense of control and hope for long-term self-regulated pain relief. Although a competent biofeedback instructor is necessary at first, he or she is merely a guide to self-help—not the bearer of relief.

Second, biofeedback may become your remedy of choice in many instances because it provides you with immediate and visible results. You don't have to display blind faith in the method or become anxious as to whether it will work. During the very first biofeedback session, the practitioner can "prove" that with a committed effort, you do have the ability to control your body's negative response to pain. This is important because, typically, pain patients have previously undergone numerous treatments, all to no avail, and come to natural medicine with amplified feelings of skepticism and a tendency to become discouraged and quit trying because they already know "nothing can help me."

To visualize why immediate, concrete results are so important to both the mental and physical aspects of chronic pain treatment, consider the golfer. Golfers don't often practice their swing without aiming to hit an actual golf ball. Although it would be easier to stay at home and practice correct stroke form in the living room (and this might actually improve their game), hitting the ball and watching the result of a particular stroke is a better way to see exactly what needs to be changed, adjusted, and practiced. In this way, golfers can be sure they're not wasting their practice time reinforcing bad habits without realizing their time is ill spent. So too with relaxation techniques that are not used along with biofeedback. You certainly can practice guided imagery, deep breathing, meditation, or other psychosomatic techniques at home and may very well break the stress/pain cycle; however, if you are practicing the technique incorrectly or if it is inappropriate for a particular kind of pain, you won't have any way of knowing that quickly without the information biofeedback provides. Practicing relaxation techniques without any way to evaluate their effectiveness can be like practicing a golf swing without a ball.

Another appealing characteristic of biofeedback is that once it is learned with the help of biofeedback equipment, you can employ the strategy at home using simply your own power of mental control. After formal biofeedback sessions are discontinued, some individuals religiously continue on the same schedule, using the relaxation techniques to maintain a healthy state of mind and body; some continue on a less frequent basis; and still others choose to set their practice sessions aside and use the skill only when they need pain relief. Many return to their practitioner for a refresher once or twice a year.

A Typical Biofeedback Session

At the first biofeedback session, you can expect a re-
markable demonstration of mind over body. The practitioner generally will ask you to discuss experiences you've already had in which your body reacted physically to a mental
image. Have you ever had the experience of imagining
something very sad—the death of a loved one, for example
—and finding yourself actually getting tearful? Have you
ever anticipated a hostile meeting with your boss or mate
and found your heart pounding at the thought of what's to
come? Have you ever replayed in your mind an aggravating
circumstance and found yourself as tense and angry as you
were when it actually happened? Well, all of these kinds of
experiences are examples of your mind affecting your
bodily responses. Hooked up to a biofeedback machine,
you actually can see evidence of your body changes in response to mental images. You might, for example, think of
an argument you recently had and find that the change in
your blood pressure or muscle tension turns on the machine's red light. Calming yourself through guided imagery
or deep breathing can turn off the light.

In subsequent sessions, the practitioner will teach you a
variety of relaxation techniques and how to use them to
attain pain relief. While practicing these methods of stress
and pain reduction, the biofeedback machines show you
your progress and reinforce your ability to ease your own
pain. In the beginning, a typical biofeedback session will
last about an hour, and you will probably be advised to
attend one to two times a week. As you become more profi-
cient in using the techniques to attain your desired level of
physical comfort, the sessions will become shorter and less
frequent.

While attending these sessions, you will be assigned
daily homework. Practicing relaxation techniques will help

you build the kind of mental strength and skill you need to combat moments of severe stress or pain when the professionally guided sessions cease and you're on your own. And at-home practice ensures maximum progress. Also, most practitioners want their patients to keep a daily log. Each day you will write down your symptoms, your sleep patterns, and your body's response to the relaxation methods you practice at home. Recording this information helps you tune in to yourself and become consciously aware of how your physical, emotional, and mental states are intertwined. This knowledge will help you gain the self-regulation skills you need to control your pain mentally.

To make your homework more interesting, your practitioner may give you some "tools" to work with. Recognizing that stress causes the body temperature in your hands and feet to drop as blood rushes to the more vital internal organs, items that monitor skin temperature can be used as minibiofeedback devices. For example, a temperature ring can help you see body temperature fluctuations caused by stress. The ring has a temperature range of 67 to 94 degrees, with little dots that light up at each point on the range. For more information about temperature rings, contact: FutureHealth, Inc., Dept. P-100, P.O. Box 947, Bensalem, PA 19020.

Stress dots also are used to monitor your body's response to stress and relaxation techniques. These stick-on dots are peeled from a piece of paper and placed on the hand. The dots change color as your hand changes from cool to warm. If you feel anxious or tense, you can practice a relaxation technique and watch the color of the dot change as you calm your stress response and raise the temperature in your hand. Stress dots can be ordered from Mindbody Inc., 50 Maple Place, Manhasset, NY 11030.

If biofeedback is an appropriate remedy for you, you should be able to see a difference in the way your body handles pain within three weeks of starting. You might actually feel pain relief, but pain relief itself is often not the first sign of success; often the rest of the body begins to normalize first and the part most affected by pain will then follow. You may find that you've developed a greater tolerance for your pain, or you might note some change in the way your body reacts to pain. If you're committed to following the program, keeping your appointments, doing your homework, and applying yourself fully, you should be off the machines and on your own after six to eight weeks from the date you start.

When choosing a health-care practitioner for biofeedback, look for appropriate credentials. Certified practitioners can be located by asking your physician for a recommendation, calling local university or hospital pain clinics, or by contacting The Biofeedback Certification Institute of America, 10200 West 44th Avenue, #304, Wheat Ridge, CO 80033.

TRANSCUTANEOUS ELECTRICAL STIMULATION (TENS)

Electrical stimulation applied to the skin has been used for the treatment of disease for many years. Only in the last twenty years, however, has transcutaneous electrical stimulation (TENS) evolved from a simple evaluative technique to a sophisticated therapeutic modality in its own right. Today, TENS is a frequently used treatment technique complete with proponents and critics as well as a wealth of literature expounding theories, opinions, and claims regarding its clinical effectiveness and its mechanism of action.

The TENS unit is a battery-operated device that delivers a low-voltage electrical current through electrodes placed on the skin. Although it isn't clear exactly why this stimulation offers pain relief, according to the *Harvard Medical School Health Letter*, there are two plausible theories. The first holds that nerves can carry only one message at a time easily. The electrical pulses from TENS overload the nerves, and the pain message shuts down. A second theory hypothesizes that the electrical pulses stimulate the body to release its own painkillers called endorphins. In a 1981 issue of *Pain*, Salar and Mingrino reported the results of their study on endorphin levels in patients without pain problems using TENS. They found that all subjects during and after twenty twenty-five-minute treatments had an increase in their endorphin levels, regardless of their basal level. This further boosts the theory of pain relief through TENS stimulation of endorphins.

Whatever the mechanism, some of the conditions successfully treated with TENS include musculoskeletal discomfort, dysmenorrhea, rheumatoid arthritis, phantom limb pain, musculoskeletal headache, and postoperative pain.

While the TENS unit is helpful in treating a variety of pain-related conditions, controversy surrounds its use. Documentation of consistently positive results has been weak, but many proponents feel there are logical reasons for this. Because pain can be very subjective, it should be understood that what works for one person may have no effect on another. Indeed, two people whose pain is caused by the same problem may need very different TENS settings to achieve the very same relief. Compounding the problem of standardizing TENS treatment for research purposes is the fact that the most effective setting varies a great deal. In many cases, it is not the TENS unit that is ineffective, but its application.

Contributing to the difficulty of accurately assessing the degree of pain relief offer by TENS is the easy accessibility of TENS units through nonprescription or other inappropriate means. After a TENS unit is purchased, its use and misuse can't be controlled. One pain patient may lend the unit to a friend who will use it improperly and without medical supervision. Units can be purchased at pawnshops, garage sales, and flea markets. TENS devices acquired in these ways are most often used by patients for inappropriate conditions and without the guidance of a trained or experienced health-care provider, hence the lack of positive results. If these patients eventually find their way to a trained doctor or therapist, they are quick to reject the idea of TENS treatment because on their own they found "it doesn't work." And with a negative mindset that will affect motivation and compliance, it may not work.

The only way to determine if TENS is an appropriate treatment for your pain is to try it under medical supervision. The initial application requires a physician's prescription. Then the unit can be bought outright (for a cost of several hundred dollars) or rented while you decide if it's effective.

TENS units offer a variety of stimulation modes to choose from. Some use "burst" stimulation, others "modulated" or "brief-intense," and still others "acupuncturelike" or "strength-duration." Your physician or physical therapist will suggest the type best for you and will apply and monitor the device, reminding you that finding the most effective use is often a trial-and-error process.

In the most common course of treatment, the physician or therapist sets the TENS device to deliver eighty to one hundred impulses a second for forty-five minutes, three times a day. This regimen is recommended based on the studies of Salar and Mingrino. These researchers found that the use of TENS triggers therapeutic endorphin levels within the first hour. After that period, stimulation may not relieve pain. Based on their findings, they recommend the use of TENS in one-hour cycles several times a day. They theorize that after the initial stimulation of endorphins for therapeutic pain relief, the endorphins become depleted. Suspension of TENS is necessary to allow the endorphin level to recover. As you become accustomed to manipulating the TENS device, you may find you need stimulation much less frequently and only in response to severe pain signals.

In addition to using TENS units for appropriate conditions with the help of trained and experienced personnel, other factors influence the effectiveness of these devices. First, remember that because of the subjective nature of pain and the interrelationship between the body and mind, the placebo effect may enhance the results (as is the case with all pain-relief modalities). Successful use of TENS also is influenced by the relationship between the patient and the therapist; you must feel confident and at ease for any pain-management therapy to give you the desired effect. And last, your motivation and willingness to participate actively in the overall treatment program will determine the likelihood of pain relief through transcutaneous electrical stimulation.

NUTRITION

The value of good nutrition may be obvious, but it is often the obvious that is overlooked. If you do not eat the right foods, the organs and cells of your body will not get the nutrients they need to function and grow properly. Since food is a basic necessity, it also has been looked upon as essential medicine from very early times. People in ancient Greece and Egypt, for example, used garlic as a cure for respiratory infections, intestinal viruses, and skin conditions. Cabbage was a remedy for ulcers and headaches. In the 1700s, English ships began to carry lemons and limes to treat scurvy, a condition that affected sailors. It wasn't until the 1900s that scientists discovered the actual substance in citrus fruit that prevented scurvy. By this time, vitamin C had been isolated from lemons, and the first fat-soluble vitamin, A, was discovered.

By the 1940s, forty nutrients and thirteen vitamins had been isolated from foods. With the 1950s and 1960s came the era of processed foods, including the booming fast-food industry. This was followed in the next two decades by numerous fad diets as people desperately tried various ways to get rid of the weight gain that comes with this convenience.

Today, it seems that the public has a greater awareness of the kinds of things they ingest. New information on the dangers of substances such as pesticides, food additives, and saturated fats—and the benefits of nutrients—have altered the way many people eat. As you revamp your diet, however, it is important to read as much as you can in order to make informed choices about what you eat. Sometimes it is difficult to discern what is the latest fad and what is sound advice. Dieticians and nutritionists can help tailor your diet to your needs if you wish to pursue nutritional therapy to treat illness or allergies, or to bolster your health.

Essential Nutrients

All food is composed of certain substances that are necessary to maintain health: fats, proteins, carbohydrates, vitamins, minerals, and trace elements. Foods are characterized by categories (fat, carbohydrate, protein, dietary fiber), and a healthy diet balances a combination of them.

Protein

Approximately 17 percent of your body is composed of protein, including muscle, hair, bone, nails, and skin. Protein is also necessary for the production of hormones and enzymes. Since protein cannot be stored in the body, it must be absorbed regularly from foods such as milk, yogurt, cheese, eggs, meat, fish, sprouts, nuts, seeds, and legumes. If you do not eat enough protein, your muscles and tissues will degenerate. Too much protein, however, could strain the liver and kidneys and disrupts the balance of minerals in your body. Protein should account for approximately 5 percent of your total caloric intake each day.

Fats

Fat is an important source of energy. It helps to maintain organs, cell structure, nerves, and body temperature. Fat also carries fat-soluble vitamins, such as A, D, E, and K, around the body. There are three types of fatty acid: *saturated fat* primarily comes from animal sources, such as meat, fish, butter, cheese, eggs, and cream; *polyunsaturated fat* comes from plant sources, such as wheat germ and safflower, corn, and sunflower oils; *monounsaturated fat* is found in olive oil, avocados, and peanuts. Saturated fats, which can increase cholesterol levels, are the worst kinds of fat to consume. Most people in our society would probably benefit from reducing their overall fat intake. Fat should constitute no more than 30 percent of your total daily caloric intake, with only 10 percent of this coming from saturated fats.

Carbohydrates

Our main source of energy is carbohydrates, which are converted into the glucose and glycogen that fuel muscles, the brain, and the nervous system. Carbohydrates come from starches and sugars. The best are starches in grains, legumes, and pastas, and sugars in fruits and vegetables. Refined sugar and flour contain high-calorie carbohydrates with little nutritional value. Unlike natural starches and sugars, which convert into glucose more slowly and are absorbed at a steady pace over time, they are absorbed quickly for instant bursts of energy. Carbohydrates should constitute the balance of your daily caloric intake (about 60 percent).

Dietary Fiber

Fiber, also referred to as roughage, is an indigestible substance found naturally in cereals, beans, nuts, vegetables, and fruits. Containing no nutrients and remaining undigested, it moves through the intestinal tract. As it absorbs liquid, it helps produce large soft stools that are easily passed. Fiber helps speed the passage of waste through the bowel and helps to remove toxic substances from the body. Low-fiber foods can take three or four days to pass through the digestive tract; high-fiber foods, in contrast, are usually passed within twenty-four hours. By consuming an adequate amount of fiber—and thus helping to move waste through the bowel more quickly—you may reduce your chances of developing colon cancer, diverticular disease, and gallstones.

Fiber occurs naturally in a wide variety of foods. Whole-grain cereals; whole-wheat, or bulgar-wheat, products; brown rice; barley; and bran are excellent sources of roughage. Legumes, oats, barley, and rye are also good sources and they form substances that restrict the amount of fat and sugar the body absorbs. This can help lower blood cholesterol levels and blood pressure. Corn, apples, carrots, brussels sprouts, eggplant, celery, potatoes, peas, and dried fruit are all good sources of dietary fiber. You should consume approximately one and one-half to two ounces (forty to sixty grams) of fiber each day.

Vitamins/Minerals

Vitamins and minerals are essential in aiding metabolism and the chemical processes in the body that release energy from food. The thirteen major vitamins are A, C, D, E, K, and eight B vitamins, often referred to as the B complex. Vitamins are soluble in either water or fat. Vitamin C and most of the B vitamins are water soluble. They must be consumed each day since they cannot be stored in the body. Any excess C or B vitamins are excreted. Vitamins A, D, E, and K are fat soluble, and they can be stored in the body's fatty tissues. Vitamin B_{12} can be stored in the liver.

Vitamins and minerals often work together and interact with each other. For example, vitamin C enhances the absorption of iron in the body. It is best to eat the daily required amounts of each vitamin and mineral in food.

If you decide to consult a nutritionist or dietician, he or she will help you devise a balanced diet and will recommend the supplements you should take according to any deficiencies you might have. If you are creating your own nutritional plan—or just modifying your eating habits—you should take a multivitamin and mineral supplement every day. This will ensure that you are getting the adequate amounts of nutrients that your body needs.

A Healthy Diet

Whole foods, or those produced with a minimal amount of processing, contain many of their original nutrients. Try to eat organically grown fruits and vegetables that have not been subject to chemical pesticides, meat and poultry that has not been given growth-hormone injections, and eggs from free-range chickens.

Generally, most people in our society need to eat more fruits and vegetables and to consume more fiber. It is best to eat fruits and vegetables raw and with their skins to ensure that you are getting all of their vitamins and minerals. Make sure to clean the skin thoroughly by scrubbing it with a brush (either a vegetable or pot-scrubbing brush) under running water to wash away unabsorbed chemicals from pesticides or other impurities. Fruits and vegetables should be eaten fresh, as they lose nutrients with age. They also lose nutrients through cooking, so try to cook them for as short a time and with as little liquid as possible. For example, if you usually boil vegetables, try steaming them instead. You'll probably enjoy their crispy texture and find that they have more taste! If you do boil your vegetables, consider using the liquid in stocks or sauces so as not to waste the vital nutrients.

Most of us also need to eat more fiber. If you now use white bread, try switching to whole-grain breads and cereals. Increase your fiber intake gradually in order to avoid a bloated feeling, which may occur temporarily.

If you want to consume less fat, eat only lean red meat in modest portions, and cook more poultry and fish. There are many good-quality low-fat products on the market, such as low-fat margarine. But use common sense in planning your diet. Remember that it is better to use just a little butter, a natural product, than to eat a lot of margarine, which contains added chemicals and hydrogenated fats.

You also should consider using skim milk and low-fat yogurt and cheese. Avoid eating rich desserts, such as ice cream or pastries, fried foods, and rich sauces.

Most of us can probably do with less sugar and salt in our diets. Refined white sugar has no nutritional value, so try cutting down your use of it. If your sweet tooth will not be denied, replace sugar with honey or fruit juices— they are natural sweeteners. Try eating fruit or sugarless baked goods and jams that are sweetened only with fruit juices.

Although some salt is necessary, most people consume too much of it since it is used in excess in many processed foods. Remember, salt occurs naturally in many foods, so there is no reason to add more. Substitute herbs and spices for salt when you are cooking, and try to eat fewer processed foods. Generally, you should consume one ounce (twenty-five grams) or less of sugar and less than one-fourth ounce (six grams) of salt each day.

It was discovered long ago that honey and salt could help preserve foods. Over the past few decades, the use of artificial additives and preservatives has increased greatly, replacing the natural ones. Some of these are harmless in small amounts, and some additives even occur naturally, such as monosodium glutamate (MSG) in fermented soy products (soy sauce). However, when restaurants add excess amounts of MSG in the preparation of food, some people experience adverse physical symptoms, such as headaches, nausea, and dizziness.

Dyes, preservatives, stabilizers, antioxidants, and emulsifiers are all food additives that can cause reactions in people who are sensitive to these substances. Most additives are thoroughly tested for safety, and they must be listed on each product, according to the rules of the Food and Drug Administration (FDA). They are not all bad, but some people are particularly sensitive to them, and they can adversely affect hyperactive children.

In order to test your own sensitivity, or that of your child, to certain additives, you need to begin a very restricted diet of bland basic foods. Gradually reintroduce one at a time those foods that are suspect and record any reactions. It is best to consult a nutritionist, naturopath, or doctor who specializes in food sensitivities when conducting a test such as this.

The best advice for planning good nutrition is to avoid foods that you know you are allergic to and to maintain a balanced diet. Eat low-fat, high-fiber, naturally sweetened foods, and let moderation and common sense be your guide.

Calorie Chart

The word *calorie* refers to a unit of energy. Calories represent the amount of energy needed to burn a particular substance. The number of calories each person needs for maximum energy depends on age, sex, occupation, and lifestyle. The following chart serves as a guide for the amount of daily caloric intake for various groups of people:

MEN

Age	Lifestyle	Calories Needed Daily
18–35	Inactive	2,500
	Active	3,000
	Very active	3,500
36–70	Inactive	2,400
	Active	2,800
	Very active	3,400

WOMEN

Age	Lifestyle	Calories Needed Daily
18–55	Inactive	1,900
	Active	2,100
	Very active	2,500
56–70	Inactive	1,700
	Active	2,000

In their quest for health, fitness, and the perfect body, many people become almost obsessive about counting calories. Remember that it is not so much the number of calories you consume, but where they come from, that is important. In other words, it is better to eat 400 calories' worth of pasta and vegetables than of ice cream. The key to planning and following a healthy diet is balance. Eat a variety of whole foods from the basic food groups, and eliminate or moderate your consumption of those foods that you know are not good for you.

Orthomolecular Medicine

Ortho is the Greek word meaning "to correct." Two-time Nobel prize–winner Linus Pauling coined the term *orthomolecular medicine* in 1968 to refer to a system of correcting the body's metabolism with the right combination of nutrients, such as vitamins, minerals, amino acids, and enzymes. All of these nutrients occur naturally in the body as a defense against illness, but sometimes the body becomes deficient in one or many of them.

In 1943, the National Resource Council's Food and Nutrition Board established the Recommended Dietary Allowances (RDAs) of various nutrients. In 1963, the Food and Drug Administration created minimum daily requirements called U.S. RDAs, which are used by food manufacturers. The levels of U.S. RDAs are based on the lowest levels necessary to prevent known diseases, such as scurvy, which are caused by deficiencies. However, these levels are not necessarily high enough to promote health and combat other common illnesses. Orthomolecular doctors and other scientists advocate setting nutritional standards not based on avoiding diseases, such as scurvy, but on promoting optimum health.

Orthomolecular medicine is holistic in that it considers mental and physical causes of biochemical imbalances in the body. Practitioners perform blood tests and use vitamin and mineral profiles to delineate levels for sixteen vitamins and thirty minerals. Many physical and mental disorders can be treated simply by supplementing deficiencies in these nutrients.

Since each individual is unique, each has different nutritional needs. People who take megadoses of nutrients should take breaks from their dosages in order to prevent overdose. Orthomolecular treatments should be supervised by a trained doctor or nutritionist.

EXERCISE

Most of us live rather sedentary lives—we drive instead of walking or riding a bike; we sit at work; and we watch television while resting on the couch. Yet exercise is vital to our physical and emotional health. It improves muscle tone and posture, increases strength and stamina, and can improve circulation and respiration. Not only does exercise reduce blood-fat levels, it can change large blood-fat globules (low-density lipoproteins) to smaller, less sticky ones (high-density lipoproteins) that move more easily and are less likely to clog arteries. Exercise also is good for the mind. It invigorates and energizes, and helps to relieve tension and anxiety. By helping to release substances that affect emotions, such as adrenaline and noradrenaline, exercise can even relieve the symptoms of depression. Have you ever heard of a runner's high? The explanation for runners' "addiction" to their exercise is that it helps to release endorphins and enkephalins, which have a mood-elevating effect. When you exercise, your body gets in shape and your mind begins to relax.

There are several different kinds of exercise, and a good workout routine should include a little of each. *Isotonic* exercises, such as weight training, stretching, and yoga, develop muscle strength and flexibility. They do not have the aerobic benefits of improving respiration and circulation, but they are essential for toning slack muscles and building strength. *Stretching* exercises, as part of your warmup and cool-down, are a must in any kind of workout.

Aerobics refers to sustained exercise that increases the amount of oxygenated blood carried to muscles and organs. In other words, any activity that increases your breathing and heart rate is aerobic: aerobic dance, step aerobics, running, jogging, fitness walking, cycling, swimming, and cross-country skiing. Stationary bicycles, Lifecycles, and StairMasters are aerobic fitness machines. When you perform an aerobic exercise, you should maintain your training-level heart rate for fifteen minutes or longer in order to receive maximum results. (See the chart on pages 128–29.) Aerobic exercise improves the respiratory and circulatory systems. It strengthens the heart muscle, makes arteries and veins more elastic, and lowers blood-fat and body-fat levels.

Anaerobic exercise is the opposite of aerobic exercise. It is characterized by short bursts of energy, such as sprinting. Although anaerobic exercise does develop muscle strength, it does not improve circulation and respiration.

When you plan an exercise regimen, consider activities

that you enjoy, that are feasible, and that you will want to do. That way you'll have a better chance of maintaining your exercise routine. Some people like to exercise alone—it is "quiet" time to think or clear the mind. Others prefer to exercise with a partner or a group because other people can be a good source of motivation and can make exercise a fun social event. You also need to consider how much time you can allot to the activity. When you have a very busy schedule, it is easy to forgo the exercising, especially if you are tired. Just try to remember that the more you exercise, the more energy you will have in the long run for all of your life's activities.

If you are over the age of forty and have been relatively inactive, are pregnant, or have a medical condition, you should consult a physician and have a complete physical exam before beginning an exercise program. When you start, begin slowly and gradually increase the duration and intensity of your workouts. Warming up is a must—stretch your muscles slowly and smoothly for at least five minutes. The endurance phase of your workout should last approximately twenty to thirty minutes, getting your pulse rate up to training-level. Cooling down is also imperative—spend five to ten minutes walking briskly and doing more stretching exercises.

The following chart will help you determine your training-level pulse rate. The resting pulse of adults is generally sixty to eighty beats per minute. To take your pulse, use the first three fingers of your hand to feel the beat in your temple or neck. Count the number of beats in fifteen seconds and multiply that by four to equal one minute.

Age	Beats per minute for Training Level
20	138–158
25	137–156

30	135–154
35	134–153
40	132–151
45	131–150
50	129–147
55	127–146
60	126–144
65	125–142
70	123–141
75	122–139
80	120–138
85	119–136

Once you get into the swing of an exercise routine, you'll probably look forward to the activities—and even feel bad if you skip a session. Remember to use common sense when you are exercising, especially if you do strenuous aerobic activity. Here are some tips:

- Do not exercise if you are ill, dizzy, or feel faint. If any of these feelings occur during a workout, cool down by walking and stretching, and then take off a day or two.

- Do not exercise if you feel severe muscle or joint pain; take a few days off and begin again gradually. If pain persists, consult a physician.

- Always warm up and cool down to avoid stiff or injured muscles.

- Allow two hours after meals before exercising.

- Avoid exercising in very hot weather and dress warmly in cold weather if you exercise outside; even if you perspire, keep all of your clothing on to avoid chilled muscles that can result in cramps or pulls.

- "No pain, no gain" may be true to a degree, but you should build the intensity of your workout gradually. Use common sense, listen to your body and mind, and don't overdo it!

CHAPTER FOUR

Arthritis

Recognized by physicians as one of the most severe chronic pain ailments, arthritis affects the lives of an estimated 11 million Americans. Often untreatable through conventional medical means, the chronic pain of arthritis reduces the sufferer's ability to perform daily tasks and negatively influences relationships with family, friends, colleagues, and even self. The annual cost of treatment and care and the losses in time, money, and productivity are colossal. These factors coupled with the frustration and depression of the disease can oftimes make the life of an arthritic patient unbearable.

But there is hope. If you have arthritis, you'll be delighted to learn that more and more often, natural medicine is being recognized as a viable and very effective treatment option. Knowing you no longer have simply to bear your pain is certainly cause for celebration—and action. Before we explain how alternative remedies can help you manage your pain, let's first take a look at exactly what arthritis is and how it damages the body.

DEFINING ARTHRITIS

Arthritis can be defined as a group of diseases affecting joints or their component tissues—but it is not a disease in and of itself. Someone may state, "I have arthritis," but the word "arthritis" only broadly describes the ailment. Analogous to cancer, arthritis exists in many forms, each with a different cause, associated pain, and treatment. If by chance a physician has told you in a seemingly succinct manner, "You have arthritis," go back and get more information regarding exactly what kind of arthritis you have.

Although there are many types of arthritis, they are commonly classified into three groups: inflammatory arthritis, degenerative joint disease, and nonarticular rheumatism. The following sections will give you an overview of each of these individually. For more information, be sure to consult a rheumatologist—an internist with special training and expertise in the various types of arthritis.

Inflammatory Arthritis

Inflammatory arthritis is a general term that by itself offers a vague diagnosis. It's simply a term used to designate a smaller subgroup of arthritis characterized by inflammation of the joint. Some specific types of inflammatory arthritis are connective tissue diseases, crystal deposition diseases, infectious arthritis, and spondyloarthropathies. These main types of inflammatory arthritis warrant a closer look.

Connective tissue diseases are a group of acute and chronic diseases characterized by involvement of joints, connective tissue, and small blood vessels. These diseases are either acquired disorders, such as rheumatoid arthritis, systemic lupus erythematosus, scleroderma, polymyositis, and vasculitis, or rare hereditary diseases, such as Ehlers-Danlos syndrome.

Rheumatoid arthritis is the most common type of inflammatory arthritis, with an estimated 3 million afflicted persons in the United States. It is characterized by the inflammation of the joints and associated structures. It is three times more common in women than in men and strikes most often between the ages of twenty-five and fifty. The finger joints are usually the first involved, followed by the hands, wrists, feet and other smaller joints. Almost all degenerations are symmetrical, affecting both sides of the body.

Rheumatoid arthritis is considered the worst of the arthritic ailments. Changes take place in the joint structures that increasingly impair and limit motion. Unless the progress of the disease is checked, it is only a matter of time before crippling deformities become permanent and severely disabling. In addition to the obvious symptoms, typical sufferers also lack energy and tire easily; they lose their appetite, lose weight, and may run a slight fever.

The process by which rheumatoid arthritis attacks the body is quite methodical and consistent. It first assaults the membrane that lines the joint (synovial membrane), causing inflammation. The inflamed membrane covers the joint and progresses into the underlying cartilage; this interferes with the ability of the cartilage to form the gliding surfaces of the joint. Simultaneously, changes occur in the bone below the cartilage; the bone loses its mineral components and becomes fibrous; the deformed material also spreads to the cartilage. As the disease infiltrates the body's system, a bloodless fibrous tissue is formed that results in stiffness in the joint.

Although brief periods of remission occur, the disease is progressive. The last and most crippling blow happens when the fibrous tissue becomes bony; this signals the end of the degenerative process. Pain and motion plateau at this time, neither increasing nor decreasing unless an outside impetus (such as a pain treatment) is applied.

The causes of inflammatory arthritis are still being researched—genetic, immunologic, infectious, and psychologic disturbances are all possible suspects. But currently there are two prominent theories. The autoimmune concept proposes that rheumatoid arthritis may be caused by an allergic reaction in which the body actually becomes hypersensitized to some part of itself. Certain abnormal substances in the blood characterize this disease in about 80 percent of patients, which provides substantial support for this theory.

Another theory asserts that the presence of an infectious agent stimulates the disease. Research findings indicate that rheumatoid arthritis may be a "slow virus" in which the symptoms do not appear until long after the virus has infected the body. However, no obvious source of infection has yet been found.

Other connective tissue diseases such as systemic lupus erythematosus, scleroderma, and vasculitis frequently are accompanied by joint symptoms that are generally not deforming. Instead, these diseases affect the body internally, involving tissue structures such as kidneys, muscle, heart, and lungs.

Crystal deposition diseases are categorized by the type of crystal involvement. The most prevalent is caused by monosodium urate. Deposits of this crystal cause gout. Gout, the metabolic disorder of uric acid breakdown, has long been associated with a violent arthritis, particularly of the toes.

Infectious arthritis is an inflammatory joint disease caused by the invasion of bodily membranes by living microorganisms, including gonorrheal, streptococcal, and staphylococcal bacteria. These usually appear following local spread of the infectious microorganism or some kind of trauma to the body. The seriousness of the disease varies considerably with the victim's age and level of resistance, the adequacy of treatment, and the nature of the invading organism.

Another group of inflammatory arthritis, called spondyloarthropathy, is characterized by the involvement of the axial (central) skeleton. Ankylosing spondylitis, Reiter's syndrome, spondylitis associated with inflammatory bowel diseases, and psoriasis are all examples of this kind of arthritis. All are believed to have hereditary origins. This group of diseases resembles rheumatoid arthritis, but is less common and is different in that it affects the central part of the skeleton rather than the exterior joints.

Degenerative Arthritis

Degenerative arthritis, degenerative joint disease, and osteoarthritis are all terms used to refer to another type of arthritic ailment. In general, degenerative arthritis is a disease of the aging process, often becoming apparent after the age of forty (although symptoms may not appear until well after the disease has a strong hold on the body).

This disease increases the rate at which the bones age. The degeneration begins at the cartilage. The gliding surface of the cartilage "flakes off." The process then destroys the binding material that holds together the bundles of cartilage fibers. We can think of the cartilage fibers as stacks of balanced pipes that had once been tied together; in weight-bearing joints these fibers soon are worn away, leaving only empty pits. Ultimately, all of the cartilage is worn away; the joint space disappears, and the bone surfaces are in direct contact. Since the cartilage is a shock absorber for the joints, arthritic pain become more apparent as the cartilage is lost. In some individuals, the cartilage wears thin by middle age; in others, it may have sustained relatively little damage at age eighty. This difference is caused by what's called the "wearing capacity" of the cartilage.

The principal symptom of degenerative arthritis is either stiffness or pain. The appearance of knobs at the end joints of the wrist and second fingers is usually the primary sign of this degenerative disease. These knobs are called Heberden's nodes and are an overgrowth (hypertrophy) of bones at the sides of the joint. Initially they are a concern to patients because of their deforming effect on appearance rather than any immobility they cause. For unknown reasons, Heberden's nodes on the fingers are nine times more common in women than in men.

Degenerative arthritis differs from rheumatoid arthritis in a number of ways. Victims of degenerative arthritis do not experience the muscular spasms or the extensive deformities caused by rheumatoid arthritis, and complete bone stiffening is quite rare. Also, degenerative arthritis causes no fever, no anemia, no loss of weight, and no inflammation of the joint membrane.

Nonarticular Rheumatism

Nonarticular rheumatism includes tendonitis, bursitis, tenosynovitis, fibrositis, and psychogenic rheumatism. This group is a potpourri of ailments that do not fall into the previous two categories. Their rate of incidence is much lower than either inflammatory arthritis or degenerative arthritis; however, they do pose a serious problem to the medical community and certainly to those who suffer their pain.

Unlike calcific tendonitis and bursitis, which usually follow a specific trauma such as muscle strain or excessive exercise, fibrositis and psychogenic rheumatism are believed to have a psychic origin and are therefore very difficult to diagnose and treat. As fully discussed in Chapter 11, these kinds of ailments are especially difficult for both patient and physician who traditionally want to find a specific physical cause for all pain and therefore put much time, money, effort, and spirit into looking for something that, in these cases, is not there. The pain of this kind of arthritis is, however, very much "there."

The challenge for those who are afflicted with arthritis is to accept the chronic nature of the ailment, turn away from short-term treatments, and look to natural remedies that are effective and safe for long-term use.

CONVENTIONAL MEDICINE FOR THE TREATMENT OF ARTHRITIS

There is no doubt at this time that arthritis is a progressively degenerative disease. Still, in our quick-results society, physicians are hounded with the urgent request, "Make the pain go away!" This certainly is one reason why conventional medicine tends to treat only the symptoms of pain and swelling. This standard treatment recently has come under scrutiny as many ask, How effective is this $10 billion industry that traditionally diagnoses and treats arthritis?

Many studies and therapeutic models have attempted to answer this question; unfortunately, the answers have been disheartening—primarily due to the conventional modes of treatment. Although comprehensive treatment programs for rheumatoid arthritis usually include rest, exercise, and various methods of joint protection, the heart of most programs hinges on daily drug use. Drug therapy has become the backbone of the conventional treatment program for two reasons: (1) It provides immediate suppression of the painful symptoms, and (2) with a yearly retail sale of an estimated $3 billion, physicians and consumers alike have come to believe that drugs are the treatment of choice for arthritis. Both of these reasons are problematic.

Most commonly, aspirin is used to reduce the inflammation of rheumatoid arthritis. In fact, the Arthritis Foundation claims it is "the most important drug for arthritis and the safest." However, it is common knowledge that high doses of aspirin over prolonged intervals can be irritating to the gastrointestinal tract and cause nausea, stomach pain, bleeding from the stomach or bowel, ringing in the ears, and decreased hearing. These results become inevitable when you consider that arthritic people must take twelve or more aspirins a day to obtain the desired anti-inflammatory results.

Another group of drugs commonly used for controlling the symptoms of rheumatoid arthritis are the nonsteroidal anti-inflammatory drugs (NSAIDs). These drugs include: Motrin, Naprosyn, Tolectin, Nalfon, Feldene, Clinoril, Dolobid, Anaprox, Advil, and Nuprin. While NSAID promotions claim they are more effective and cause less gastrointestinal upset than aspirin, the physical repercussions of chronic use are staggering.

Many studies have shown that NSAIDs have serious and irreversible side effects. One study has estimated that 20,000 hospitalizations and 2,600 deaths each year can be linked to NSAID use in rheumatoid arthritis patients. More specifically, other studies have shown the link between these drugs and the development of bleeding ulcers. Even the Food and Drug Administration (FDA) is convinced of the harmful effects of these drugs. According to an FDA press release: "200,000 cases of gastrointestinal bleeding, with 10,000 to 20,000 deaths, occur each year due to the 68 million prescriptions of non-steroidal anti-inflammatory drugs, or NSAIDs, used for arthritis." Subsequently, the

FDA strengthened the NSAID warning label to read: "Serious gastrointestinal toxicity such as bleeding, ulceration and perforation can occur at any time, with or without warning symptoms, in patients treated chronically with NSAID therapy." Certainly long-term drug therapy with NSAIDs is not a safe approach to the management of arthritis pain.

In addition to aspirin and NSAIDs, corticosteroids are widely prescribed to reduce the inflammation of arthritis. These drugs are more powerful than aspirin and NSAIDs, but they also have more negative side effects.

The body quickly develops tolerance to these drugs, so the dosage is repeatedly increased to attain pain-relief results. Unfortunately, large doses of a corticosteroid such as cortisone can cause harmful complications. When injected directly into the joint over a prolonged period of time, this drug eventually may cause joint destruction, just as surely as will the disease itself. When taken orally, the short-term benefits are heavily outweighed by the long-term side effects. Users become vulnerable to infection, peptic ulcer, diabetes, or high blood pressure, and lose calcium in their bones, which can then spontaneously fracture. The Arthritis Foundation recognizes these possible consequences yet asserts that despite the dangers and drawbacks, in special cases the use of these hormones is necessary. Perhaps that is true, but certainly only a very rare circumstance would call for exposure to these horrendous side effects over the implementation of natural therapies proven safe and effective.

In cases of crippling arthritis where drugs have become ineffective, conventional medicine offers another, more invasive, option—the implantation of electrodes in the brain. Electrical brain stimulation releases the body's natural painkillers, endorphins, and can in many cases reduce or even eliminate the pain of arthritis. (See page 20 for a complete discussion of electrode use.)

Unfortunately, long-term use of electrodes brings disappointment to many users. The body can build up a tolerance to the stimulation of the electrodes. When this happens, users find themselves using higher and higher voltage levels more and more frequently with diminishing results.

Finally, some people with arthritis turn to surgery. The primary reasons for surgery are joint repair, joint replacement, and removal of the joint lining. In many cases patients seek surgery to remedy the pain and correct the cosmetic deformities caused by the disease. The implantation of artificial knuckles in patients disfigured by rheumatoid arthritis, for example, is becoming quite popular, as is hip replacement surgery. Still, as all arthritis sufferers learn, this disease is progressive and not curable.

Even after drug therapy, electrode implantation, and/or surgery, the pain of arthritis returns. At this time of complete frustration many people come to realize the value of natural remedies as a part of their pain-control program for arthritis. Self-management skills are the best way to maximize any benefits gained from the conventional therapies and, in addition, will help forestall the disease progress and maintain continued physical and mental health.

NATURAL MEDICINE
FOR THE TREATMENT
OF ARTHRITIS

There is a fundamental difference between the way conventional medicine deals with arthritis and natural medicine's remedies. Allopathic medicine confronts pain by imposing some kind of external device or remedy into the treatment program; proponents of natural medicine believe that the key to pain management is held within the body itself. The following discussion focuses on different types of natural remedies and their effectiveness as pain relievers for arthritic patients. Be sure to read the full description of these remedies in Chapter 3.

Acupuncture

Many studies have shown that acupuncture is highly effective in treating the pain of arthritis. In particular, one study led by Dr. Bruce Pomeranz, a neurophysiologist at the University of Toronto, indicates that while both acupuncture and electroacupuncture can relieve any type of arthritic pain, electroacupuncture seems especially potent in the treatment of osteoarthritis. (See pages 41–47 for a complete discussion of acupuncture.)

Acupressure

Acupressure has been found to be an effective therapy for the pain of arthritis. Its application is most helpful for relieving the pain accompanying nonarticular rheumatism (myofibrosis and fibrositis). Most patients with this kind of arthritis suffer from "tender points" on their body; acupressurists devote their energies to these points.

Acupressure also is used as an alternative treatment of rheumatoid arthritis to reduce the inflammation that accompanies the disease. There are many points on the body that, when stimulated, increase circulation, reducing inflammation and increasing joint mobility.

Acupressure is an especially appealing remedy because it can be self-administered. A trained acupressurist can teach you how to locate your tender points. You also can be trained to treat yourself by reading a good self-help book on the subject. As a sample, you might try applying firm pressure each day to the following potent points; just hold each point firmly for about two or three minutes or massage gently. (If you find that your hand is too weak to apply finger pressure for this long, you can use the knuckles or your fist or even a golf ball or small rock.)

Problem Area: arthritis of the wrist, hand, fingers, and bones of the hand

Li 4: in the webbing between the thumb and index finger at the highest spot of the muscle when the thumb and index finger are brought close together

TW 4: in the depression on the back of the wrist, from the base joint of the fingers, move straight back to the center of the wrist

P 7: on the palm side of the wrist, in the depression in the middle of the wrist crease, between the two tendons

Si Ferg: on the palm side of the hand, in the center of each skin crease on the second through fifth finger joints closest to the hand

Ba xie: in the four forks where the hand meets each finger

Problem Area: elbow and shoulder

Li 11: on the upper edge of the elbow crease

Problem: headaches, insomnia, stiff neck, neck pain, fatigue, and general irritability

GB 20: below the base of the skull, in the hollow between the two large, vertical neck muscles, two to three inches apart depending on the size of the head

Most people with arthritis will have to practice these self-acupressure techniques two to three times a day for six months and continue once a day for prevention and health maintenance.

In addition to the points just mentioned, other arthritic locations (such as the hip, ankle, and knee) can benefit from acupressure. Be sure to consult a practitioner and ask about your particular pain.

Botanical Medicine

The herb feverfew often is recommended as a natural remedy in the treatment of arthritis. Feverfew contains analgesic as well as anti-inflammatory properties that are most helpful in treating arthritic joint pain.

Exercise

Exercise is helpful in managing arthritis pain. Exercise moves the blood flow to the affected joints and keeps them flexible. It increases the oxygen available to promote mineral absorption by the bones. Stretching exercises ensure that the joints move smoothly, and strengthening exercises maintain muscle tone. The specific exercises that are best for you depend on the type and severity of your arthritis as well as your overall physical condition. You and your health team should work together to build an exercise program to meet your ability and needs.

Some Recommended Exercises

Swimming is a particularly good type of exercise for people with arthritis. Water exercise involves most of the typical calisthenics you do on land. However, the buoyancy of

the water supports your muscles and joints so that you feel
lighter and able to move easier, and you run less risk of
injury than if you were performing the same exercises on
land.

If you can't swim, walking might be a beneficial exercise.
Walking has been found to slow the spread of the disease,
maintain proper body weight, and improve flexibility for
many arthritis sufferers. Although exercise can't completely
stop the progressive nature of the disease, walking will help
you stay limber and enable you to remain active.

Try the following specific exercises for localized areas.

For Fingers   To help increase movement in the joints
of the fingers, start with joint one at the tip of the finger.
Slowly bend it with the other hand until you can reach joint
two. Continue gradually applying pressure through joint
three. You can reverse this process, starting with joint three
and working up. Do this exercise as many times in the day
as feels comfortable, but at least once a day.

For Wrists   To increase flexibility and movement in
the wrists, place palms together with fingers interlaced.
Slowly apply pressure by pushing the palms together on
one side and then the other. Push to the point of discomfort, then just a little bit beyond. Repeat as many times as
feels comfortable, but at least once a day.

For Elbows   Place palms and fingers together, bringing arms to right shoulder. Now press downward on a diag-
onal toward your left knee, straightening both arms. Go
slowly and push just a little beyond any discomfort. Repeat
on the other side. Repeat as many times as feels comfortable, but at least once a day.

For Shoulders Clasp your hands behind your neck. Slowly pull your elbows as far back as you can, then bring them forward and touch them together if you can. This exercise rotates your shoulders to help increase movement and also stretches out your chest muscles. Repeat three to five times.

For Calves and Ankles

1. Using a stable object such as a table or wall, lean into the object with both hands. Bend your left knee as you lean forward and stretch your right leg behind you, straightening the leg as much as possible. Make sure both feet are pointed straight ahead to get the right stretch. You should feel a good stretch in your calf if your heel is as flat to the floor as possible. Hold for twenty seconds. Switch to other side and repeat with left leg.

2. Now place both legs back together as you lean into the table or wall. Slowly raise up on the balls of your feet and back down, pushing your heels flat to the floor. Repeat ten times. This exercise is excellent for promoting flexibility and movement in the calves and ankles.

Homeopathy

The use of homeopathy in the treatment of arthritis is generally complex, requiring professional guidance. Homeopathic treatment for rheumatoid arthritis requires expert care, with special attention to diet and exercise. Homeopathy for chronic osteoarthritis also requires expert care. For isolated flare-ups professionals often prescribe the following remedies to be taken four times daily for up to two weeks. (However, no treatment should be undertaken without consultation with the appropriate medical personnel.)

- Use *Rhus tox. 6c* for pain relieved by heat but aggravated by cold and damp; it may be more insistent when resting but wears off with continued movement; stiffness is often worse in morning.
- Use *Bryonia 6c* for severe pain made worse by heat and movement and often relieved by cold applications.
- Use *Pulsatilla 6c* when heat makes joint pains worse and brings on feelings of weepiness.
- Use *Calcarea phos. 6c* when affected joints feel cold and numb; pain and stiffness increase with weather changes; you may feel weakness when climbing stairs.
- Use *Ledum 6c* for aftereffects of steroid injections, or for small joints, especially toes, that give pain and make cracking noises; effective for joint pains that seem to progress up the body and pain that is relieved by cold application.
- Use *Arnica 6c* for joint pains caused by, or made worse by, injury.
- Use *Aconite 6c* for severe flare-ups in cold or dry weather.

Hydrotherapy

Hydrotherapy is a standard treatment for arthritis. Many patients find relief from the pain and stiffness through heat and/or cold therapies. Some patients find that soaking in a warm bath or using a heating pad relieves their symptoms; others swear by the therapeutic effect of ice packs and cold water soaks. You'll have to experiment to find the remedy that is most beneficial for you.

You also might want to try a combination of the two. A contrast bath lets you use heat to increase circulation and cold to reduce swelling in one therapy session. You use a contrast bath by soaking the inflamed joint in warm water, then in cold water, and then in warm water again. You repeat this cycle every three to five minutes for a total of twenty minutes.

Hypnosis

Hypnosis is most effective in controlling pain that is psychogenic in origin. Therefore, fibrosistis and psychogenic rheumatism are treated quite effectively with hypnosis.

Hypnosis is also a recommended therapy for pain that is exacerbated by stress, tension, or anxiety. Although most types of arthritis have a specific organic root, some patients have noticed a connection between the degree of pain they feel and the tension in their life at the moment. If your arthritis pain seems to be aggravated by stress and is responsive to relaxation therapies, it may well be treated through hypnosis.

Nutrition

All forms of arthritis are affected by poor nutrition. To begin nutritional therapy, you need to remove pollutants from your body that increase the body's acidity and leave behind waste materials. The most harmful pollutants are caffeine, alcohol, and nicotine. Coffee, alcohol, and cigarettes leave waste in the body that must be cleaned up by white blood cells. Rather than attend to their regular duty of maintaining good health, these cells are overtaxed and their efficiency is weakened when they must spend their energies cleaning out the debris left behind by these substances. If you find yourself addicted to alcohol, coffee, or cigarettes, talk to your doctor about how you can best break the habit to begin your nutritional therapy.

Nutrition and Inflammatory Arthritis

As new bone cells generate, their health is based on the amount of nutrition the body provides. If your body is lacking in minerals, for example, the generation of new bone cells is weakened. This malnourishment problem is the core of arthritis. When we are malnourished, contaminated wastes caused by excess acidity in the body feed the new cells. This causes inflammation that later becomes some form of arthritis.

To stop the cycle of deterioration, you must reduce the amount of waste that's in the bloodstream (by reducing your exposure to pollutants), and you must increase the amount of nutrition in the bone. Bones need the minerals calcium, magnesium, phosphorus, and manganese and the vitamins C, E, and K. They all perform like a team; they must be present in the correct balance before the bone structure and the cells can develop correctly.

Green vegetables most effectively remedy the nutritional deficiencies that cause and aggravate inflammatory arthritis. These vegetables supply the six nutrients necessary to remedy arthritis, and they also magnetize the removal of waste from the body. Chlorophyll, which gives green vegetables their color and content, is of the same exact molecular structure as the hemoglobin in the human blood—except that the center molecule of chlorophyll is magnesium, while the center molecule for hemoglobin is iron. Because it is magnesium (derived from the word "magnet"), it magnetizes impurities into the chlorophyll and out of the bloodstream. So green vegetables perform double duty: They increase nutrition at the greatest level possible and they clean impurities out of the bloodstream.

The color of green vegetables indicates how valuable they are: The darkest greens of kale, watercress, parsley, chard, and mustard greens are most nutritious. The medium group includes spinach and lettuce. And the lower end of the groups includes cucumbers and celery, which have high water content and low chlorophyll.

Degenerative Arthritis and Nutrition

Degenerative arthritis (osteoarthritis) responds well to the same nutritional therapy described for inflammatory arthritis with emphasis on mineralization. Minerals are accepted into a cell through a transfer that must occur in an oxygen environment, but poor nutritional and health habits interfere with the body's oxygen supply. This can cause or negatively affect osteoarthritis. Diets high in fat and sugar content make proper mineralization doubly difficult. Not only don't they bring minerals into the body, they leave debris that smothers the current oxygen supply around the cells.

Lack of exercise also decreases mineral absorption. If you avoid exercise because of your arthritis, you're denying your cells the oxygen they need to absorb minerals and improve your condition.

To use nutritional therapy as a treatment for degenerative arthritis, you should try the following.

- Eliminate pollutants such as coffee, black tea, cigarettes, and alcohol.
- Eliminate foods high in fat and sugar content.
- Begin a supervised exercise program.

• Ask your doctor for advice about increasing your intake
  of the minerals calcium, magnesium, phosphorus, and
  manganese, and the vitamins C, E, and K.

Nonarticular Rheumatism

Nonarticular rheumatism does not involve the bones,
but rather affects the arteries and nerves. Because the arteries and nerves are made vulnerable to pain sensations by
poor nutrition and the wastes left by pollutants, you can
treat this condition by improving your diet. However, nutritional therapy is not as effective as the structural manipulations provided by chiropractors and osteopaths.

Nonarticular rheumatoid conditions such as fibrositis
and psychogenic rheumatism that are considered psychological in origin often can be treated successfully through
nutritional therapies such as those described in Chapter 11.

Popular Nutritional Therapies for Arthritis

Food allergies play a major role in the development and
support of arthritis. Many arthritics seem particularly sensitive to the nightshade family of vegetables (tomatoes, eggplant, red pepper, and potatoes). These certainly are not
"bad" foods, but they are acidic. The body may become so
accustomed to reacting negatively to junk food with high
acid levels that it reacts impulsively to these chemically
healthy, but acidic, foods also. Therefore, arthritis sufferers
may want to avoid the nightshade vegetables.

Don't treat your arthritis with gold salts. Gold salts take
away the pain of arthritis by readjusting the mineralization
of the body. But in the long run they weaken the body,
increasing the problem and the pain.

Nutritional therapy will never reverse bone contortions caused by arthritis. But if you alkalize and nourish your body long enough, nutritional therapy can end your struggle with arthritis. Over 70 percent of the people who use this approach experience dramatic recovery in less than one year.

Psychotherapy

Cognitive-Behavioral Therapy

Arthritis sufferers often develop pain behaviors and attitudes that interfere with pain management. If you find that you reward your pain by resting in bed or avoiding daily tasks and responsibilities, and if you often think about how your pain is ruining your life and causing you to miss out on things that you'd like to do, cognitive-behavioral therapy can help you manage your pain. This kind of psychological therapy will help you identify those thoughts and behaviors and replace them with positive ones that put you in control and reward pain management thoughts and actions.

Couples/Family Therapy

Along with cognitive-behavioral therapy, family therapy is an effective approach to pain management. Family members are involved in your pain in two ways:

1. They enable you to continue your negative pain behaviors by taking over your responsibilities, catering to your pain, and giving attention to your moans and groans.

2. They escalate your stress response by words and actions that imply you are sometimes lazy, hypocondriacal, and in essence a "pain" to live with.

Therapy that involves family members allows all of you to see and react to pain in a different way, and to voice your feelings about pain in a safe and constructive environment.

Relaxation Techniques

Stress has been found to aggravate arthritis. When you're upset, angry, anxious, or depressed, your muscles tense, your breathing becomes shallow and faster, and the blood flow throughout your body is restricted. All of these physical stress reactions can increase your pain. Learning to calm the stress response can help you manage your pain. The following relaxation exercises are suggested as natural remedies for arthritis; be sure also to read the full discussion of relaxation and its effect on pain on pages 91–107.

Guided Imagery and Meditation

While the ability of even deep meditation to ease the pain of arthritis may be short-lived, it's still a useful technique because you can perform this therapy anytime and anywhere.

One type of meditation proven especially helpful uses guided imagery to create "movies of the mind." These are short ad-libbed meditations that can reduce pain temporarily. The technique helps you visualize your joints as healthy and nonpainful in an attempt to "trick" your brain into producing sensations of calm and comfort.

Here is an example of a movie of your mind that you might try:

My hands are healthy and strong. They're beautiful, smooth, calm hands. They are healthy and pain-free. I can move them easily one finger at a time. The first finger bends smoothly and easily. The next finger also moves without pain or stiffness. Each of my fingers is happy to take its turn moving. First one, then the next, then the next. Then they all move together. Without pain I can move my fingers and use my hands to do whatever I want. I can open bottles; I can hold my toothbrush; I can comb my hair. My hands do whatever I want them to do.

Autogenic Training

Autogenic training can be used to relieve the pain of arthritis. It enables you to focus your attention on particular parts of your body without putting any physical pressure on your inflamed joints.

Deep Breathing

Deep-breathing exercises are effective in stopping the body's stress response. This gives you the ability to control the muscle tension that can trigger your pain.

Progressive Muscle Relaxation

Progressive muscle relaxation *is not recommended* for arthritis sufferers. Intentionally tensing muscles around inflamed joints can worsen joint pain.

Biofeedback

Biofeedback has been found to be especially helpful in easing the stress-related pain of arthritis. Psychologist Jean Achterberg-Lawlis has published encouraging results about her use of biofeedback in the treatment of arthritis. In one study, a group of arthritic individuals diminished the amount of pain they were feeling, reduced the tension created by the pain, and in general slept better. In another study, one group of arthritics had biofeedback training and another had a standard physical therapy program. Not only did the group using biofeedback and relaxation feel better, but an erythrocyte sedimentation rate (ESR) blood test measuring the activity of the disease showed that the immune system had held stable against the disease or the arthritis had abated.

TENS

Transcutaneous electrical stimulation often is used to ease arthritis pain. It has been found to be especially helpful in reducing pain that is localized in a specific joint. Full benefits sometimes take some experimentation. Your physical therapist or doctor will help you try different positions and levels of stimulation until you hit on the best combination.

Arthritis is a very unpredictable disease characterized by flare-ups and remissions. Without warning its pain strikes, and just as suddenly it may disappear. This very nature of the disease makes evaluating the full effectiveness of natural remedies difficult and may sabotage your efforts.

Consider the person who faithfully follows a natural remedy course of pain control and then experiences a sudden exacerbation of symptoms or, conversely, improves when not complying with the self-management regimen.

The natural course of the disease may lead this person to the wrong conclusion about the effectiveness of the therapies and cause him or her to give up too soon. This is a shame; the premature rejection of potentially useful remedies robs this person of the full benefits that can be gained with commitment and perseverance.

Don't make the mistake of giving up too soon. Experiment with a number of different therapies; focus on ones that fit your lifestyle and needs, and then work hard and consistently to reach your dream of living an active and productive life despite your arthritis.

CHAPTER FIVE

Lower Back Pain

The numbers are staggering. Seventy-five million Americans suffer from back problems, with 7 million new sufferers arising each year; 1.5 million of these new cases are totally disabled either permanently or temporarily. In the workplace, the numbers are equally surprising. According to the National Safety Council's "Accident Facts":

- Back injuries account for at least 20 percent of all occupational injury cases.

- Such injuries account for about 22 percent of all reported or compensated work injuries.

- They account for some 23 percent of cases involving disability, meaning some 400,000 disability cases occur each year at work.

- Average costs per back injury in a year have been estimated at close to $4,500 in wage compensation and almost $1,600 in medical payments, compared to some $3,400 and $1,300 respectively for all other parts of the body.

These numbers indicate that millions of Americans need a detailed understanding of how the back operates, what causes their pain, and what methods of treatment are most appropriate and beneficial.

THE BACK

The spinal column is a complex support system comprised of bone, muscle, nerves, tendons, ligaments, disks, joints, and cartilage. In addition to support, it provides the body with strength and stability along with movement and flexibility. The spinal column also houses the spinal cord, the nerve cable that links the brain to the rest of the body.

The spine is made up of cube-shape bones called vertebrae. The first seven vertebrae stemming from the head are known as cervical vertebrae. These support the head and allow it to turn, extend, and flex.

The next region is the thoracic vertebrae, which support the arms and shoulders. These twelve vertebrae are also part of the body's rib cage, providing protection to the heart and lungs. They are larger than the cervical vertebrae because of the extra weight they support.

The lumbar or lower back section allow for forward- and backward-bending motion. These five vertebrae are the largest because they support the most weight.

The sacral vertebrae are a series of five fused bones wedged between the hip bones.

Finally, the four coccyx bones are a series of very small vertebrae that aid the pelvic bones in supporting the powerful buttock muscles.

A healthy back has a number of notable characteristics. It normally curves in four places: at the sacral region, the lumbar region, the thoracic region, and the cervical region, creating a "double-S" curve. In addition, muscles up and down the spine work together in a balanced fashion with pressure distributed evenly throughout the spinal curves. Any alteration in this arrangement can cause one section of the spine to overcompensate for the other, leading to a weak and fatigued spinal structure. This occurrence causes or compounds back problems.

VERTEBRAE AND DISKS

The approximately thirty-three vertebrae that make up the spine have bony protrusions known as spinal processes that help form the housing for the spinal cord. These protrusions also have ligaments that interlock each vertebra, allowing for movement.

Between the vertebrae lie yet other structures called disks. Within the disk is a gelatinous fluid known as nucleus pulposus. This fluid, together with the vertebra and the cartilaginous disk, acts like a shock absorber. When pressure is applied, the fluid is compressed. When pressure is relieved, the fluid springs back to its normal shape. This action is crucial to healthy vertebrae because without it they would grind together, eventually causing complete deterioration.

Damage to the disk can cause fluid to escape, which would put pressure on nerves surrounding the vertebrae. These nerves lead to the body's longest nerve—the three-foot-long sciatic nerve, which runs from the lower back down to the foot. The pain emanating from pressure placed on the sciatic nerve is known as sciatica.

CAUSES OF BACK PAIN

Because the spine is a complex collection of interlocking pieces, back pain can arise for a variety of reasons. Sometimes the root of the pain is found in degenerative or hereditary disease. Other times, in fact in the majority of cases, the pain involves biomechanical stresses caused by obesity, improper lifting, poor posture, injury, age, or a sedentary lifestyle.

Degenerative and Hereditary Diseases

Some back pain is caused by disease. The most common organic causes of back trouble include herniated disk, anklosing spondylitis, spondylolithesis, metastatic disease, and degenerative disk disease.

• Herniated disk: The spinal disks are located between the vertebrae and act as the body's shock absorbers. The soft core of each disk is covered by a layer of fibers. A disk becomes herniated when the core ruptures through this layer. The result is a shooting pain down the leg accompanied by back pain.

• Anklosing spondylitis: This disease is a form of inflammatory arthritis that most commonly afflicts males (5 to 1) between the ages of twenty-five and thirty-five with a family history of this problem. The early symptoms come and go without much notice, but over the years the spine becomes increasingly rigid.

• Spondylolisthesis: This condition is caused by a defect in the spinal arch that results in the sliding forward of one vertebra onto the one below it.

• Metastatic disease: This term refers to a disease that spreads from an afflicted point to other parts of the body— in this case, the back. The back pain is really a secondary symptom of disease somewhere else.

• Degenerative disk disease: This disease, which is not completely understood, is caused by the aging process and causes pain and disability.

Biomechanical Stresses

Less than 10 percent of lower back pain has an organic origin. Instead, most often the pain is caused by conditions called biomechanical stresses, which overload the spinal structure. Motion ultraviolet film shows in glowing detail that all the pressure of the body falls on the lower back. With proper posture and care, the back adapts well to this burden. However, when posture is poor, or the vertebrae are twisted or strained, back pressure pushes on nerves, causes unbalanced hip structure, and twists disks and vertebrae. With 65 to 75 percent of the population walking around with poor upper spinal posture, it's no wonder that lower back problems are so common.

In addition to the natural pull of gravity and poor posture, the following biomechanical stresses frequently cause lower back pain:

- Compressive forces from improperly lifting a heavy weight
- Tension on ligaments and muscles from bending forward in an extreme position
- Twisting forces from exposure to abnormal positions over a long period of time
- Trauma from a fall
- Weakening or atrophying of muscles and pressures on disks from a lifetime of poor posture
- Static muscle strain from long periods in uncomfortable positions (sedentary workers are especially prone to this)
- Muscle spasm from injury
- Tense, painful muscles from a distressed emotional state

- Tight, short muscles from heavy manual labor

- Improperly fitted shoes (especially high heels!)

These biomechanical stresses are the source of most chronic back pain and are the ones most likely to be remedied by natural therapies.

CONVENTIONAL MEDICINE FOR THE TREATMENT OF LOWER BACK PAIN

Back pain is an extremely common complaint in doctors' offices all over the country. Whether you take your pain to a family practitioner or an ortheopedist, your treatment regimen will probably begin with a series of diagnostic tests.

Diagnosis of Back Pain

Diagnostic tests look first for serious disease and disorders. If these can be ruled out, other tests can sometimes pinpoint the source of the pain.

Tests typically prescribed include the following:

- X rays are used to eliminate any probability of disease, inflammation, abscess, or other bone disorders.

- Myelography is used to find muscle spasm and soft-tissue damage such as swelling. This procedure is a type of X ray in which a contrast dye is injected into the spinal fluid space.

- A diskography is a process similar to myelography in which the injected dye demonstrates the integrity of the disk.

- Electromyography (EMG) is a procedure in which a very thin needle-type electrode is inserted into the muscle to electrically measure the nerve and muscle integrity as well as the muscle's ability to contract and relax.

- A computerized axial tomography (CAT) scan is a type of X-ray scanning procedure that enables a doctor to see more closely and in greater detail any soft-tissue damage.

Other diagnostic tests might include magnetic resonance imaging (MRI) and thermography.

Once the cause of your back pain is determined (as nearly as possible), the physician has a variety of treatment procedures to choose from.

Drug Therapy

Painkillers are most commonly used to manage back pain. Over-the-counter analgesics and nonsteroidal anti-inflammatories usually are the first line of treatment. Although they do ease the perception of pain, muscle relaxant tranquilizers (such as Darvon and Percodan) also are usually prescribed to relieve the muscle tension in the lower back. In the acute stages of back pain where there is a recurrence of spasms and mobility is severely inhibited, the anti-inflammatory drugs, analgesics, and muscle relaxants or any combination of the three often are very helpful in managing the pain.

However, in the case of *chronic* back pain, drug therapy should be considered a dangerous treatment approach. As detailed in Chapter 1, the negative side effects of long-term drug use are far too physically and mentally disruptive for drugs to be used for anything other than temporary relief of acute pain.

Nerve Blocks

Two kinds of nerve blocks are used most frequently to treat back pain: Trigger-point injections place a local anesthetic at the actual site of pain to block the nerve impulses carrying the pain message, and injection of a steroid into the epidural space surrounding the spinal cord and nerves blocks the pain signal from traveling.

Although these blocks sometimes can help relieve postural stress and allow a back-pain patient to participate in beneficial exercises, relaxation techniques, and other natural rehabilitative treatments, nerve blocks are inappropriate for long-term treatment. Because the relief lasts only as long or slightly longer than the effects of the anesthesia, the injections require habitual and inconvenient outpatient care. Also, trigger-point injections treat only the symptom of pain and not the cause; the pain always will return. Moreover, because a trigger-point injection can aggravate the condition, often the pain returns with more intensity than before. And finally, the body can develop a tolerance for the anesthesia, requiring more frequent injections with reduced effect.

In addition to these problems with injections, in the October 3, 1991, issue of *The New England Journal of Medicine,* researchers showed that the injection of steroids into the joints in the backbone provides no significant benefit.

Surgery

Approximately 350,000 spine operations are performed in the United States each year, but there is a growing consensus in the medical community that only a small fraction of these people actually needed surgery or will benefit from it.

Back surgery is a possible option for those suffering from back pain in only two situations: if there is a tumor or ruptured disk placing pressure on the major nerve root or the spinal cord, or if there is spinal cord or nerve root compression from a fracture or other major instability such as traumatic injury.

Diskectomies, spinal fusion, and laminectomies are the most commonly performed surgeries for these conditions.

A diskectomy removes a ruptured or herniated disk. The success rate is only 40 to 80 percent, and subsequent disk surgeries are significantly less successful.

Spinal fusions are performed to stabilize the spine or straighten the abnormal curves caused by scoliosis. Vertebrae are "welded" together by bone grafts that are placed between the vertebrae. In time the vertebrae and the bone grafts will heal as a single piece.

In a laminectomy, the surgeon cuts through a part of the bony ring (the lamina) surrounding the spinal cord or nerve roots in order to remove a herniated disk. Laminectomy is near the top of the list of unnecessary operations. Of the 200,000 such surgeries performed each year, experts at the Rand Corporation (a research think tank) estimate that up to 40 percent, or 80,000 operations, are unnecessary. Up to 70 percent of patients with a herniated disk will improve without surgery. And according to follow-up studies done up to ten years after back pain was diagnosed, patients who had surgery fared no better than those treated medically.

Other Conventional Forms of Treatment

Four other treatment approaches to back pain are used to remedy disk problems: percutaneous diskectomy, administration of chymopapain, traction, and braces or corsets.

Percutaneous diskectomy involves removal of portions of a damaged disk. In this controversial procedure, a needle is introduced into the disk and disk material is sucked out.

In 1982 the Food and Drug Administration approved the use of chymopapain in the treatment of spinal problems. Chymopapain is derived from the papaya plant and is chemically related to the active substance in meat tenderizers. This substance is injected into the disk space to dissolve the problem disk.

Traction frequently is used as a conservative treatment in an effort to avoid surgery. Traction is used to straighten and stretch the soft tissue around the joints in order to straighten the spine. This aids in pulling the vertebrae slightly apart, allowing a herniated disk to heal.

Braces or corsets often are suggested to support and immobilize the spine. These form-fitting jackets are most helpful for elderly patients or for patients who need some support after surgery. Braces are problematic only if the patient becomes dependent on them and relies on this artificial support and avoids back exercises that are necessary to naturally strengthen the muscles around the spine.

NATURAL MEDICINE
FOR THE TREATMENT OF
LOWER BACK PAIN

Too often conventional medicine treats chronic lower back pain in ways that are invasive, costly and/or addictive, and unfortunately frequently unsuccessful. The following

natural therapies offer a more holistic approach to back
pain that addresses the cause and offers preventive therapies, maintenance tactics, and pain-control remedies.

Chapter 3 presents a complete discussion of how and
why these natural therapies work to relieve chronic pain.
Be sure to read this chapter before you talk with your
health professional about implementing any of the following remedies.

Acupuncture

Acupuncture is highly effective in treating lower back pain.
A trained and experienced acupuncturist can restore the
body's natural flow of energy and interrupt the sensation of
pain. In addition, treatment will be geared to resolving underlying energetic imbalances that have resulted in lower
back pain.

Oriental medicine recognizes many causes of low-back
pain. The low back is ruled by the kidneys. When Oriental
medical practitioners refer to an organ, they are not referring to something that is identical to the organ named in
Western medicine. The Oriental organ includes energetic
functions in addition to physiological functions. These energetic functions have mental and emotional components
and have an affinity to certain seasons, colors, and climates.
In Oriental medicine, the kidneys are the root of all the yin,
yang, and essence (or *chi*) in the body. And, like a savings
bank, much of what we have is stored in the kidneys. As we
age, the amount in storage declines. As the kidneys become
more deficient, we can begin to suffer low-back pain or
become susceptible to low-back injury. Since the emotion
associated with the kidneys is fear, living in fear, or sudden
fear, can injure the energetics of the kidneys. On the other
hand, having kidneys that are weak can cause unexplained

feelings of fear. Since the kidneys are especially sensitive to cold, being exposed to cold can contribute to weakness of the kidneys. In addition, imbalances in diet, such as drinking lots of coffee, can injure the energetics of the kidneys, as can overwork or excessive sexual activity.

Of course, there are other causes of low-back pain besides those that are kidney related. For example, traumatic injury can cause *chi* or blood stagnation. An acupuncturist will treat you differently depending on the cause and the quality of your pain.

Acupressure

When your hip hurts or your lower back aches, your body compensates by shifting the burden off that area and placing it on another. Unfortunately, this only compounds back pain. Acupressure relieves the pressure and helps the back muscles relax, causing the vertebrae to fall naturally into alignment. In addition, since acupressure utilizes the same acupoints as acupuncture, therapeutic effects of regulating *chi* and blood flow result.

You can self-administer acupressure by applying firm pressure each day to the following potent points. If you have a weak back, these points may be very tender. In this case, several minutes of light touch instead of deep pressure can be most effective.

B 23/B 52: between the second and third vertebrae of the lower back at two points: at one and a half and at three inches away from the spine at waist level

Benefits: Relieves lower backaches, sciatica, pelvic tension, hip pain, and tension.

CV 6: two finger widths directly below the navel

Benefits: Relieves lower back weakness, tones weak abdominal muscles, and prevents a variety of lower back problems.

B 40: in the center of the back of the knee crease

Benefits: Relieves low-back and leg pain, knee pain, back stiffness, and arthritis in the knees, back, and hips as well as muscle cramps.

GV 26: directly below the nose at its midpoint where it meets the trough above the upper lip (Stimulate the point while gently bending backward and forward.)

Benefits: Relieves back pain that is centered on the spine.

The effectiveness of acupressure can be enhanced by a healthy diet and some lifestyle changes.

Botanical Medicine

The herb *Salix alba* taken from the white willow bark is an analgesic that may offer relief for lower back pain. Other analgesic herbs include passionflower, hops, and valerian. If the pain also involves inflammation, you might ask your doctor about trying feverfew as well.

Chiropractic

There is now compelling scientific evidence that chiropractic manipulation is effective in the management of both acute and chronic mechanical low-back pain.

Chiropractors first will determine the cause of the pain through a series of diagnostic tests such as X rays, CAT scans, or straight leg raises. If nerve-root compression is present (as with a herniated disk), the practitioner may choose to use other forms of treatment, such as traction tables or other traction devices.

When the cause of pain is found to be muscle-based, a chiropractor can work on the specific vertebra involved, manually moving one segment at a time to bend, twist, or stretch the vertebral joint and help to reposition it. The Palmer trial published in a major medical journal, *Manual Medicine*, supports the use of chiropractic to treat lower back pain. This trial related to chronic patients who had experienced lower back pain for an average of three and a half years. After receiving chiropractic adjustments two or three times a week for two weeks, both objective and subjective measures showed significantly greater clinical improvement in the experimental group than in the control group.

In general, four weeks of treatment are required before improvement can be observed. Chiropractors often use a variety of natural remedies to complement the spinal manipulation. They may recommend acupuncture, massage, exercise, and diet changes. All these work in harmony to ease lower back pain.

Exercise

Because bed rest decreases disk strain and prevents aggravation, it is a preferred treatment for acute back pain. Indeed, rest can hasten recovery from simple backache due to strain of muscles and ligaments, and it is especially appropriate for backache caused by ruptured disks or nerve damage. But even in these cases, bed rest can be overdone and always should be considered a temporary remedy.

Because chronic back pain is not a temporary condition,

bed rest is never the whole solution. In fact, it is often a large part of the problem. Extended bed rest weakens the body's natural ability to fight off pain and rehabilitate painful areas. Just two weeks of forced bed rest deconditions muscles and can result in a loss of vertebral density of up to 7 percent. This deterioration cannot be expected to cure lower back pain. Instead, movement—exercise—can restore back function.

Exercise performs a variety of services in the treatment of lower back pain. Among them, consider that exercise:

- contributes to weight loss, which reduces stress on the spine (Every additional pound you weigh adds ten pounds of stress to your back.)
- strengthens muscles to prevent pain caused by strain
- relaxes tense back muscles to ease existing pain
- prepares back muscles for the trauma of surgery when necessary and promotes quick recuperation and rehabilitation

In September 1989, *The Physician and Sports Medicine* magazine printed a story about Joe Montana, quarterback for the San Francisco 49ers, that offers a good example of the benefits of exercise for treating back injury. In 1986 Montana had a bulging L4-5 disk. His surgeon prescribed an off-season rehabilitation program that allowed him to be active without stressing his spine. Later during a regular season game, Montana herniated the disk and developed additional bulging at the L4 and L5 levels. One week after the injury, Montana underwent bilateral laminectomy with bilateral disk excision and decompression of the spinal stenosis.

Within three days of surgery, Montana was in the gym using Nautilus equipment. Within ten days, he was walking rapidly. Eight weeks after surgery, Montana played his first game. Surgeons believed his rapid recovery and rehabilitation was possible because his off-season exercises had put him in great shape to undergo surgery and come out of it quickly.

Montana's rehabilitation will be a lifelong process. Sometimes that's the drawback of exercise as a natural remedy for back pain—it isn't a quick fix or a one-shot deal. Montana's surgical consultant says, "If [Montana] lets himself go, he'll get weak and stiff, which will put pressure on his back. The segment of his back that was injured will deteriorate and will require further surgery." Exercise therapy requires a commitment to continue a program that will build up the muscles of the back over time.

The kind of exercises recommended for back pain varies according to the patient's needs. Stretching exercises build up flexibility; abdominal strengthening exercises reduce strain on the back; extension exercises stretch and strengthen the back if the muscles were injured by bending; and aerobic exercise increases the supply of blood to the nerve root, changing its metabolism, promoting healing, and possibly preventing further injury.

The following set of exercises can be used to increase lower back strength and flexibility. But before you begin any exercise program, remember that exercise therapy needs to be implemented gradually on a progressive schedule. What is best for you and your pain condition should be judged and supervised by a physician, pain-clinic staff member, or physical therapist.

Exercise #1: Stand on your right leg using a wall or sturdy piece of furniture for support. Grasp your left ankle with your left hand behind your back and pull gently, stretching your thigh. Hold for thirty seconds. Repeat on the other side.

Exercise #2:   While in bed, or on a flat surface, keep your knees bent, bring your left knee to your chest for fifteen to thirty seconds; in the meantime, straighten your right knee. Repeat, bringing your right knee to your chest and straightening your left knee. Bring both your knees to your chest for thirty seconds.

Exercise #3:   Lie on your stomach for a few seconds to a few minutes. Prop yourself up on your elbows for a few seconds to a few minutes. As your flexibility increases, press your back farther upward with your hands and forearms. Keep the pressing time brief. Repeat ten times.

Exercise #4:   Begin by sitting on the floor and putting your left leg out in front of you, toes straight up, and then swing the left leg over as far as possible toward the left side. Bend your right knee and bring the right heel in close to the crotch, keeping the left knee flat on the floor and holding your left hand in the small of your back. Sitting as erectly as possible, twist to the left until you're facing the outstretched leg. Now reach out your right hand and try to touch your left toes, bending from the hips. Hold there a few seconds for a slow, steady stretch and return to the original position. Repeat. Next, switch legs and stretch to the right side.

Exercise therapy often is combined with hydrotherapy and massage for maximum benefits.

Homeopathy

Homeopathic treatment of back trouble caused by tension and stress requires expert care. However, the following homeopathic remedies are often prescribed for the treatment of some back problems. (However, no treatment should be undertaken without consulting with the appropriate medical professional.)

For lumbago pain, specific remedies to be taken four times daily for up to ten days:

- Use *Bryonia 6c* for pain that comes on in cold, dry weather and is made worse by slightest movement; the back feels bruised and sensitive to slightest touch.
- Use *Nux 6c* for lumbago aggravated by movement or a chill.
- Use *Aesculus 6c* for lower back pain aggravated by walking and stooping.
- Use *Rhus tox. 6c* when the lower back feels stiff and bruised, especially after resting and in damp, cold weather, and moving around reduces pain and stiffness.
- Use *Dulcamara 6c* for pain aggravated by stooping and by exertion followed by exposure to cold and damp.
- Use *Rhododendron 6c* when lumbago is worse before a thunderstorm or in dry, cold weather.
- Use *Sulfur 6c* when there is violent stitching pain on stooping, aggravated by movement and especially bad at night in heat of bed.
- Use *Cimicifuga 6c* when lumbago causes restlessness and prevents sleep.

For coccyx pain, specific remedies to be taken three times daily for up to seven days:

- Use *Cicuta 6c* for recurrent tearing or jerking pain.
- Use *Kali bichromicum 6c* for pain that gets worse when sitting down or walking.

- Use *Hypericum 6c* for pain brought on by a fall.

- Use *Causticum 6c* when the coccyx feels bruised and aching, and improves in damp, wet weather.

- Use *Silicea 6c* when pressure and drafts increase pain and cause constipation.

- Use *Antimonium tart. 6c* when the coccyx feels as if it has a heavy, dragging weight attached to it.

For sciatica, specific remedies to be taken every hour for up to ten doses, or every thirty minutes if pain is acute:

- Use *Colocynth 6c* when pain shoots down the right leg to foot, causing occasional numbness and weakness; pain seems worse in cold or damp weather.

- Use *Rhus tox. 6c* when there is tearing pain, relieved by heat and gentle movement, but aggravated by inactivity, cold, and damp.

- Use *Arsenicum album 6c* for sciatic pain in an invalid or elderly person that is worse at night and aggravated by cold; it improves with gentle exercise.

- Use *Lycopodium 6c* for pain in the right leg, aggravated by pressure and lying on the right side, most severe between 4 and 8 P.M.

- Use *Kali carbonicum 6c* for burning pains shooting into the knee and foot, aggravated by coughing; leg feels itchy; pain is especially bad around 3 A.M.

- Use *Magnesia phosphoricum 6c* for lightninglike pains in the right leg that are soothed by heat and aggravated by coughing.

- Use *Gelsemium 6c* for burning pains that are especially bad at night, preventing sleep, and also bad after rest or as you start to walk.

Hydrotherapy

Hydrotherapy is a standard mode of treatment for the relief of back pain. The decision whether to use cold or hot water therapies, however, should be determined by your physician.

Cold water therapies are generally used to reduce the inflammation caused by acute injury. Cold restricts blood vessels and reduces the amount of blood flowing into the injured area, thus reducing swelling.

Hot water therapies are most appropriate for chronic conditions. Heat increases blood flow, improving circulation and thus supplying more oxygen and nutrients to the area. It also speeds the flow of the body's natural painkillers, endorphins, to the site. In addition, heat eases the muscles tension so often responsible for lower back pain. Hot towels, heating pads, or hot baths all can be used to soothe spasming muscles.

Hypnosis

Hypnosis is particularly effective in easing back pain that is exacerbated by muscle tension. Through hypnosis deep states of relaxation can be attained, allowing tense muscles to relax and blood circulation to flow smoothly.

Hypnosis also can be used successfully to help a person suffering degenerative or hereditary back problems dissociate from the pain. Dissociation can be used to control pain by separating the area of pain from the rest of the body. Hypnosis can lead a patient to believe that the back pain is not debilitating. Or he or she may be able to displace the pain sensation to a smaller, less vulnerable area of the body. Hypnosis can block awareness of pain by altering its perception, and it can even promote amnesia to help patients forget their periods of pain.

Although hypnosis does not work for everyone due to varying levels of suggestibility, it is a therapy worth trying as a natural remedy for chronic back pain.

Massage

Massage often can ease back pain caused by trigger-point tension. Muscles are arranged in bundles of fibers, and these bundles are covered by a glistening white membrane called the fascia. At times, and for reasons we really do not understand, local areas of muscle and fascia knot up, become inflamed, and cause the rest of the muscle to contract and go into spasm. Sometimes nerves become trapped between these contracting muscles, and this pressure on muscles and nerves causes radiating pain.

These knots can be flattened by careful manipulation of the trigger point. You might try this common at-home remedy for relief from the pain of knotted muscles:

Have your partner place his or her thumb directly over the knot and, with a circular motion, flatten the knot. He or she may have to roll it back and forth for about two to three minutes, but eventually the knot should disappear. It's not necessary to exert too much pressure on the knot; the length of time spent on the knot rather than the force exerted is what does the trick.

Deep breathing during the process should help; inhale before the pressing, and as your partner presses, exhale slowly. With the knot's disappearance should come at least temporary freedom from the stiffness and the soreness of the trigger-point pain.

Nutrition

For Disk Problems

Proper nutritional therapy combined with exercise sometimes can improve bone density and repair degenerative disk problems. Complete recovery is not very common, but for some people nutritional therapy does work and for many others it offers varying degrees of pain relief.

Because disk growth occurs from the outside inward, disk degeneration looks like a tooth with cavities eating at its structure. To remedy this circumstance, you want to absorb through the bloodstream different minerals that will recalcify the outer disk. These minerals include phosphorus, magnesium, manganese, and calcium. Sources of these minerals in the vegetable group are collard greens, mustard greens, broccoli, brussels sprouts, and cabbage.

For Pain Caused by Biomechanical Stresses

The base of the spine is the part of the body most directly nourished by our food intake. Therefore, nutritional therapy can improve the strength and health of the spine very effectively to prevent further injury and also to relieve and even eliminate your current pain.

A healthy spine needs a rich supply of vitamins A, D, E, and K, and also the minerals silicone, manganese, calcium, and phosphorus. These nutrients can be readily found in the following:

- all green vegetables
- root vegetables such as sweet potatoes, yams, and jicima

- squash, especially hubbard, acorn, and butternut
- grains, especially buckwheat, millet, and quinoa

Along with adding nutrients to your body, it's important to eliminate the nutrient destroyers you may be ingesting. These include coffee, black tea, cigarettes, alcohol, processed foods, and meats.

By changing your diet, you can become pain-free.

Psychotherapy

Quite often back pain as a physical condition is difficult to diagnosis precisely and treat. One primary reason for the difficulty is the number of psychological factors that may be involved. Patients complaining of low-back pain often are influenced by depression, job dissatisfaction, drug or alcohol abuse, and the prospect of workers' compensation, to name a few. In addition, the placebo effect seems to be particularly strong for low-back pain. In one psychological evaluation of back pain, one-third of the patients reported marked relief of back pain after receiving treatment they did not know was only a salt water solution.

Because of this close relationship between back pain and psychological factors, psychotherapy is strongly recommended as an integral part of a pain-management program. Exploratory psychotherapy, psychoanalysis, and Gestalt therapy can help patients uncover the root cause of stress, anxiety, or depression that may be finding its release in back pain.

Couples therapy and family therapy also is often useful in the treatment of back pain. These kinds of therapies help family members understand the psychological factors involved in back pain and teach them how they may be enabling the pain to continue by unintentionally reinforcing pain behaviors.

Behavioral and cognitive therapy also is used quite frequently to treat patients with back pain. In fact, many behavioral psychologists use operant conditioning techniques for patients who seem resistant to other forms of treatment. This approach to behavior modification rewards desirable behaviors and ignores undesirable ones. One behavioral approach uses exercise, rather than drugs or rest, as a reward for back-pain patients. Patients work toward a specific, attainable exercise goal, such as a given number of repetitions or amount of time on an exercise bicycle; they stop when the goal is attained. This method makes rest (the reward for exercising) dependent on the exercise itself, and not on the experience of pain or fatigue.

Reflexology

Reflexology has been known to ease the pain of an aching back. Although the art of reflexology is quite complex and requires professional administration or more self-help training than can be offered here, you might try these few simple massage points:

- To reduce general spinal pain, massage the inner part of the arch a few inches up from the heel on both feet.
- A sore coccyx or tail bone can be remedied by massaging the inner arch just a few centimeters up from the heel.
- Sciatic pain requires a vigorous massage of the heel of the right foot.

Relaxation Techniques

Lower back pain can be controlled with relaxation techniques. Because we often are unaware of our daily tensions,
we can exacerbate and prolong back pain without realizing
it. We grow tense and our muscles contract, constricting
the blood flow. Pain sets in. More circulation is cut off,
creating a vicious circle. There's more pain, more tightening, more stiffness. A regular routine of relaxation techniques can stop this cycle and ease the pain you now feel
and prevent back pain in the future.

Guided Imagery

Movies of the mind used in guided imagery are a most
effective way to stop back pain. They are most powerful if
you concentrate your images of healing action on a specific
location. In a typical scene, you might imagine in your
mind:

> *I see the affected area receiving fresh blood and oxy-
> gen. I can see my muscles growing stronger and more
> resistant to pain. I am feeling pain-free. My back is
> strong and healthy.*

In addition, guided imagery allows you to administer a
mental massage to the painful area. Imagine firm pressure
kneading out the pain and replacing it with soft, supple,
and pain-free muscles fibers.

You can use these mental images in your mind for dual
action against back pain. Play them to prevent pain when
you're in a tense situation, and use them to lessen the degree of a current pain attack.

Meditation

Meditation begins with relaxation. It requires you to empty your mind of all noxious thoughts and sensations. Meditation allows you to combine the healing effects of guided imagery, deep breathing, and distraction while you create within your body a chemical and emotional balance. Yoga therapy is particularly beneficial to sufferers of back pain because the yoga postures alone promote healthy spinal positions.

Progressive Muscle Relaxation

Progressive muscle relaxation can be especially useful in controlling lower back pain. This technique teaches you to recognize muscle tension in various parts of the body and consciously relax the tension at will. Because back pain often is caused or accompanied by tense back muscles, this therapy allows you to control this source of pain.

Other Techniques

There is a strong connection between chronic back pain and muscle tension caused by stress. Therefore, relaxation techniques that reduce stress can ease lower back pain. In addition to the techniques just described, autogenic training, distraction, music, and laughter all have been applied successfully to back-pain relief. Try a variety of these therapies and choose just a few to use as a routine component of your pain-management program.

TENS

Transcutaneous electrical nerve stimulation (TENS) can produce some relief in over 30 percent of patients with intractable back pain. This is an impressive therapeutic result, considering the therapy is not invasive nor risky. Certainly, TENS is a remedy to be employed before a patient considers drug therapy or surgical treatment. Ask your physician to tell you more about the use of TENS in the treatment of back pain.

CHAPTER SIX

Migraine Headaches

There is little debate that headaches are the most prevalent and costly pain disorder of our age. Frequent and severe headaches are experienced by an estimated 45 million sufferers in the U.S. alone, causing untold personal and financial losses. In 1992, a special newsletter edition of *USA Today* reported that headache sufferers lose 157 million workdays a year and industry loses $50 billion annually in absenteeism and medical expenses associated with headache.

The prevalence of headaches can be attributed primarily to the abundance of stress that we all experience in our daily lives. Indeed, the headaches that nearly everyone gets once in a while are aptly named tension headaches because they are brought on by tension and stress, more often than not. This condition involves the actual tensing or mechanical contraction of the muscles in the region of the head and neck. The pain of a tension headache can be felt in areas such as the shoulders, neck, head, and jaw.

The tension headache can be classified as either chronic or episodic. Chronic tension headaches are those that occur more than fifteen times each month for more than six months, or occur more than 150 times each year. Episodic headaches are those that occur less often. The root of each, however, is the same: tension.

Most tension headaches are managed effectively with

over-the-counter analgesics. However, the long-term use of any drug is potentially harmful physically and is inadvisable; that's why tension headache sufferers can and should learn to control their pain with natural therapies. The variety of relaxation techniques and modes of psychotherapy explained in Chapter 3 all can be used effectively to help patients manage their stress and, at the same time, substantially reduce (if not eliminate) the intensity and frequency of tension headaches.

Tension headaches can be quite painful and even chronic, but they should not be confused with migraine headaches—the subject of this chapter. The debilitating and recurring pain of migraine headaches has far more complex roots, symptoms, and treatment plans.

DEFINING MIGRAINES

Migraine is a type of vascular headache caused by overstrained blood vessels in and around the head. The intensity of migraine pain can impair one's ability to concentrate and focus on even the simplest task, affecting work production, quality of life, and, of course, physical health. A recent study in *Patient Care* reports that the migraine headache is one of the most common neurological disorders, affecting as many as 17.6 percent of women and 5.7 percent of men in the United States—a total of 23.6 million people. Although migraines are not yet fully understood by the medical community, years of research on this subject have uncovered some interesting facts.

• Migraines affect three times more women than men.

• The severity of the pain does not differ by sex.

- Migraines can begin during childhood, but most often begin during adolescence and certainly will appear before age forty.
- Migraines often run in families, although no specific genetic link has been found.

The physiological process that causes migraines is well studied and understood. The process begins when the arteries and arterioles constrict. This constriction decreases the amount of blood able to reach the brain. When this happens, the body attempts to compensate for the reduced blood flow. The brain stimulates the production of neurochemicals that are intended to maintain adequate blood flow and proper nutrition to the cells of the brain. Many times the brain "panics" and stimulates an overabundance of these neurochemicals. This in turn causes the dilation and swelling of particular blood vessels, especially around the temples, forehead, and eyes, continuing the chain reaction by stimulating stretching in the vessel walls. This series of actions, which is the brain's way of compensating for the reduction of the blood supply, produces the sensation of pain.

SYMPTOMS

Although the symptoms and pain of migraine tend to vary from one person to the next, they do present a number of general characteristics. Some people experience a migraine with an aura (often called a classical migraine). As the blood vessels constrict and reduce the blood supply to the brain, many people get a "warning" that a migraine is coming. This warning, or aura, presents itself through a collection of physical symptoms such as tingling or weakness of the limbs, dizziness, or faintness. Also, the aura commonly affects vision; sufferers either will see things that aren't there, such as sparkling lights or zigzag designs, or they will be blinded by shimmering lights that block their vision completely.

Others experience a migraine without aura (sometimes called a common migraine). The pain for both is the same.

The pain of a migraine is confined to one side of the head (the word "migraine" actually means "one side of a head") and can be described as a throbbing or pounding centered around the eye and/or temple. The pain lasts from four to seventy-two hours and may be accompanied by nausea, vomiting, and a heightened sensory perception that makes lights, sounds, and smells seem stronger and more irritating than usual. The pain of migraine usually is aggravated by moving or bending over.

TRIGGERS

A most common question from migraine sufferers is "What causes this?" Unfortunately, there is no one easy answer. The external stimuli that trigger migraine headaches are many, and patients often find that they are susceptible to different ones at different times.

Stress is a common migraine trigger in two ways. A migraine attack may occur smack in the middle of a stressful experience, such as a traffic jam or argument. Or it may occur as a let-down response when the stress subsides and the body is ready to relax.

There are a number of other common causes as well. In some women, migraines are associated with hormonal factors such as menstruation, menopause, oral contraceptives, pregnancy, and postmenopausal therapy. Medications can trigger a migraine headache; these include nitroglycerin, hydralazine hydrochloride (Apresoline), and reserpine. Certain foods have become associated with migraines including chocolate, cheese, red wine, processed meats, foods containing monosodium glutamate (MSG), or NutraSweet artificial sweetener. Also, temperature changes, vigorous physical exercise, and hypertension all can spark an attack. Even seemingly benign things such as heat, fatigue, flickering lights, glare, fluorescent lights, and strong smells of perfume or gasoline can cause migraines.

Pinpointing the specific cause of your migraine can be difficult because triggers often act in combination with each other. For example, you may show no reaction to cheese or red wine, but if you have the two together after a stressful day—BINGO, it's migraine time. Another person may eat Chinese food for years without any problem, but if he eats a Chinese dish containing MSG on the day after losing a night's sleep, this could trigger a migraine. Some migraine sufferers have successfully zeroed in on their triggers by keeping a written log of their activities, diet, and experiences on the days they suffer migraines. This is very helpful in managing migraines. If you can identify what causes your attack, you can limit recurrences by avoiding your triggers.

CONVENTIONAL MEDICINE FOR MIGRAINE

The conventional approach to the treatment of migraine (or any headache, for that matter) is typical of most modern medical therapies: Treat the symptoms. In this case, physicians find that headache pain is most responsive to medication. Aspirin and other over-the-counter nonsteroidal anti-inflammatory drugs (NSAIDs) such as ibuprofen are usually suggested and do offer some mild temporary pain relief.

Prescription medications also are used with varying degrees of success. Commonly prescribed prescription analgesics include meclofenamte (Meclomen), naproxen (Anaprox), and indomethacin (Indocin). These medications are generally effective in blocking the sensation of moderate to severe pain, but they also are known to cause negative side effects.

Muscle relaxants also are used in the treatment of migraine headaches. These prescription drugs are considered effective in muscle-contraction headaches and are believed to provide relief in the early stages of a migraine. Commonly prescribed muscle relaxants include carisoprodol (Soma), chlorzoxazone (Parafon Forte DSC), metaxalone (Skelaxin), orphenadrine (Norflex), cyclobenzaprine hydrochloride (Flexeril), and methocarbomal (Robaxin).

For increased analgesic effect, some pain-relief drugs are combined with caffeine, aspirin, or even codeine. It is the general consensus in the conventional medical community that these combination analgesics (including Norgesic, Robaxisal, Equagesic, Fiorinal, and Tylenol #3) are the most effective treatment for the pain of migraines.

Unfortunately, despite the welcome pain relief it offers, drug therapy should not be used for long-term treatment of any pain condition (as explained fully in Chapter 1). Because migraine is a chronic condition, habitual use of drug therapy may begin the abysmal cycle of drug tolerance requiring increased dosage and thus potential negative side effects. Analgesic rebound headaches are a typical example of why drug therapy may be an inappropriate treatment for chronic pain. When analgesics are taken frequently, the body adapts to the continual presence of the pain reliever in the system. When the analgesic effect begins to wear off, the awareness of pain becomes even greater. That's why those who choose drugs as their primary source of pain relief may be increasing the disruptive effects of migraines. Analgesic drugs, both over-the-counter and prescription varieties, also are known to cause gastric irritation and ulcers and therefore should be used only on a temporary basis and with caution. Add to this the potential addiction problem characteristic of muscle relaxants, and it becomes clear that migraine sufferers need to explore alternative treatment options as a supplement to traditional methods.

NATURAL MEDICINE FOR MIGRAINE HEADACHES

Natural medicine takes a holistic look at the problem of migraine headaches. By reestablishing a healthy flow of energy through the body and mind, the root cause of the migraine is addressed and the frequency and intensity of migraine pain is affected. Be sure to read Chapter 3 for a complete discussion of *how* each of these remedies works to ease chronic pain.

Acupuncture

Acupuncturists believe migraine headaches are caused by an imbalance in the body's flow of energy. They use acupuncture to reestablish this equilibrium, thereby treating the cause and the pain of migraine.

Although acupuncture can ease the pain of an attack, migraine is best treated with this therapy in a preventive approach.

Before treating a client who comes presenting with headache, an acupuncturist will want to determine several key facts, including the location of the headache. Because the head is traversed by many meridians, the location of the headache determines which meridian(s) is involved. For example:

• Pain in the occiput and nape of the neck indicates blockage in the bladder meridian.
• Pain at the forehead and above the eyes indicates the stomach meridian.
• Pain by the temples and side of the head is related to the gallbladder meridian.
• Pain at the top of the head indicates an imbalance in the liver meridian.

Each of these headaches is relieved by applying acupuncture to different points.

In addition, the acupuncturist will want to know what the pain is like, if it is associated with particular weather patterns, food intake, time of day, and so on. As a result of determining this, the acupuncturist will be able to design a treatment program to restore the flow of *chi* to normal and prevent the recurrence of headache.

Acupressure

Acupressure can be used as an adjunct therapy in the treatment of migraine pain and the underlying cause of this physical disturbance. If you want to self-administer acupressure, try using these points:

GB 20: the base of your skull in the hollow areas on either side of the vertical neck muscles, two to three inches apart depending on the size of your head

Slowly tilt your head back with your eyes closed,

and firmly press up with your thumbs underneath the skull for one to two minutes as you take long, deep breaths.

Lv 3: on the top of your foot in the valley between the big toe and second toe

Using either your thumb or your right heel, apply pressure on top of this spot and rub for one minute. Then switch and work the opposite foot.

For headaches on the forehead and above the eyes:

Li 4: in the webbing between the thumb and index finger at the highest spot of the muscle when the thumb and index finger are brought close together (Use in combination with Lv 3 to relax the jaw.)

For headache on the sides of the head or temples:

TW 5: on the forearm, three finger widths above the wrist crease, between the two bones

Botanical Medicine

Many herbal medicines claim to dull the symptoms of migraine headache. One especially has received quite a bit of attention from the National Headache Foundation. This herb is called feverfew and is being used extensively in England for the prevention of migraine attacks. Despite the fact that most headache experts in the United States regard the use of feverfew as experimental, the National Headache Foundation has reported recent findings that continually taking feverfew extracts decreases the occurrence of migraine headaches in certain individuals.

Chiropractic

There is clear evidence that chiropractic treatment is effective in the management and cure of both common and classical migraine. Perhaps the most thorough prospective study of patients in chiropractic practice is that by Wight published in the *ACA Journal of Chiropractic* in 1978. This reviews earlier studies since 1923, which report success rates (cure or marked improvement) between 72 and 90 percent. Wight's success rate in a well-designed study of eighty-seven consecutive patients was 74.7 percent. This success rate was maintained two years after treatment ended, and the improvement rate applied equally to common and classical migraine and for male and female patients.

Another study, known as the Parker trial, after the principal researcher, was commissioned and funded by the Australian Federal Government expressly to determine whether chiropractic adjustment provided an effective treatment for migraine. It found that it did. The eighty-five patients in the trial had suffered regular migraine attacks for an average of nineteen years. They were divided into three groups: one receiving chiropractic adjustment, one medical/physiotherapy manipulation, and one medical/physiotherapy mobilization. All three treatments proved to be effective, but the chiropractic results indicated superiority on all measures reported—complete cure, frequency of attack, mean duration, mean disability, and mean intensity of pain.

The evidence of general effectiveness of chiropractic treatment is now compelling. A reason for this effectiveness seems to be that stiffness and pain in the cervical spine is a frequent and major factor. Ten years ago it was unusual for a medical practitioner to refer a migraine patient for chiropractic care. Now it is becoming more common.

Exercise

Although continuous and strenuous exercise actually can be the cause of a migraine headache, it is believed that as a prophylactic tool, a moderate aerobics program can lessen the frequency and intensity of the migraine when it occurs. This belief is based on the fact that exercise is known to ease body tension and improve circulation; both of these physiological changes reduce the likelihood of migraine attacks.

Indeed, migraine sufferers who are placed on a regular aerobics training program cut the frequency of their headaches in half. Try this: Walk and/or run for thirty minutes a day, three times a week. As your body readjusts over several months to the increase in oxygen, nutrients, and fitness level, you may experience a reduction in your migraines that echoes the study results that have concluded: "The fact that headache frequency significantly decreases following aerobic training suggests that it suppresses some trigger mechanism related to this disorder."

Homeopathy

Homeopathic practices often have been found to relieve the pain of migraine headaches. There are several popular remedies, but each is unique to the specific characteristics of the individual's pain, and therefore it is difficult to offer generalized therapies. Those most commonly used in the treatment of migraine pain are belladonna, bryonia, and nux vomica. You should consult a qualified professional about taking any of these remedies.

Belladonna commonly is used to treat the violent, throbbing pain of migraine that is aggravated by light, noise, touch, strong or unusual smell, or motion and is characteristically worse in the afternoon. Belladonna is the most commonly prescribed homeopathic medicine for headaches associated with high fever and is unique in that it suits headaches relieved by sitting or made worse by going down a slope or stairway.

Bryonia is best used to treat the steady ache of migraines that are severely aggravated by motion. Sufferers who cannot even make slight motions with the head or eyes without increasing the pain's intensity are likely candidates for this homeopathic remedy. Bryonia commonly is suggested for the treatments of headaches that are worse in the morning and are accompanied by nausea and vomiting.

Nux vomica commonly is suggested for the treatment of migraines caused by overeating, alcohol, coffee, other drugs, or fatigue. It also frequently helps those sufferers who feel especially irritable.

Hydrotherapy

The advice to take a shower when a migraine strikes may sound like a brush-off, but actually it is a technique with proven results. Neurologist Augustus S. Rose, M.D., of the UCLA School of Medicine, says that contrast therapy has helped many of his migraine patients. To try contrast hydrotherapy, take a cold shower followed immediately by a hot shower, and then cold to hot again.

Hypnosis

Hypnosis can influence the pain of migraine headaches in two ways: It can reduce the frequency of migraine attacks by training the body to deal with personal stress triggers, and it can reduce the patient's perception of pain when a migraine does occur.

Whether you seek the help of a professional therapist

trained in hypnosis or learn self-hypnosis by reading books, this alternative remedy has been found to be very effective in managing the pain of migraines.

Massage

A good neck and shoulder massage can relieve the muscle tension caused by stress, and it can improve circulation inhibited by constricting vessels. Both of these changes can ease the pain of mild migraine headaches.

A massage professional can administer Swedish massage for either prophylactic or therapeutic pain relief. You also might prevent the onset of a migraine by practicing this simple massage routine each day:

First, let your head droop forward, and then turn your head from left to right as far as you can. Then let your head slump forward and begin massaging the back of the head and neck with firm pressure in slow, rhythmic patterns.

Nutrition

There is little doubt among the experts that the root of many people's migraine headaches is in their diet. In fact, in some cases migraines can be classified as a food allergy. While each migraine sufferer needs to do some detailed detective work to uncover the particular food that serves as a trigger, it can be done, and the results have been astonishing.

Studies such as the 1983 report on migraine headaches by Dr. Egger and his associates in London consistently support the view that there is a link between the foods we eat and the frequency of migraines. Egger studied eighty-eight children who suffered from frequent and severe migraine headaches. The children were put on a diet that slowly eliminated foods associated with migraines and their symptoms were monitored. Amazingly, 93 percent of these children suffered no migraines so long as they avoided the foods to which they were allergic.

Food found to be closely linked to migraine headaches include: milk and other dairy products, chocolate, cola drinks, corn, onions, garlic, pork, eggs, citrus fruits, wheat, coffee, alcohol (especially red wines and champagne), cheese (particularly aged or cheddar), chicken liver, pickled herring, canned figs, and the pods of broad beans. In addition, two common food additives whose suspected link to migraine headaches deserves attention: monosodium glutamate (MSG) and nitrates. These additives may be present in almost any processed food, but are found most notably in hot dogs, bacon, ham, salami, and the like. As a migraine sufferer, it is very important that you begin to read food labels and avoid foods containing these additives.

Migraines also can be caused by an intestinal disorder (perhaps as many as 50 to 60 percent!). Poor nutritional habits can severely disrupt the level of healthy bacteria found naturally in the gastrointestinal tract that are absolutely necessary to good health. Although all the bacteria you'll ever need for a healthy gastrointestinal tract throughout your life are supplied in the first few moments of breastfeeding, the things you take into your body after that time can wipe them out, causing a whole array of health problems—including migraines. Healthy bacteria are destroyed by processed, unhealthy foods, by pollutants such as caffeine, alcohol, and nicotine, and most especially by the many antibiotics we take.

As a migraine sufferer, you need to increase your intestinal flora by changing your diet. To begin, it's important to reduce the level of acidity in your body because in order to reproduce themselves, healthy bacteria need an alkaline environment. You should eliminate pollutants such as coffee, black tea, cigarettes, and alcohol. You also must reduce your intake of acid-based foods such as meats, cheese, white breads, and processed foods. Replace these foods with those having a high pH level such as vegetables, fruits, grains, and beans.

Next, you need to add bacteria to your gastrointestinal tract. There are six bacteria in the intestinal tract and all six must be consumed together. (Some natural health advocates recommend acidophilus alone, but one bacterium cannot remedy the problem.) Go to a reputable health food store and look in the cooler section for a product that contains all six of the naturally occurring bacteria. Several companies in the United States make this available in powder or capsule form.

Once you return the bacteria count in your gastrointestinal tract to normal, you may find your migraines will disappear.

Psychotherapy

Because migraine headaches can be caused or aggravated by stress, a variety of psychological therapies can be helpful in reducing the frequency and intensity of these headaches. All require the help of a professional therapist.

Cognitive Therapy

The way you think about your pain influences your experience of it. Cognitive therapy can teach you to think about your migraines in ways that can raise your pain threshold, thereby diminishing the debilitating aspect of this condition.

Cognitive therapy also can help you change the way you think in general. Often negative thoughts can intensify the body's response to common daily stresses. A therapist can help you deal with stress and perhaps eliminate your migraine trigger.

Behavioral Therapy

Behavioral therapy is an appropriate approach for migraine sufferers who have developed pain behaviors in response to this disorder. Common pain behaviors include chronic complaining and worrying, incessant talking about the migraine experience, developing dependent or helpless attitudes, withdrawing from social activities, and anticipating migraines at every turn of the day. A therapist can offer concrete steps that can help you overcome these habits and give you a more positive and active role to play in your own pain management.

Other kinds of psychotherapy including couples, family, supportive, exploratory, psychoanalysis, and Gestalt also have helped migraine sufferers find the root of their pain and deal with its presence in their lives.

Reflexology

The practice of reflexology can be used to ease the pain of migraine headache. The fleshy underpart of the big toe is the area of the foot believed to relate to the health of the neck area. Vigorously massaging the underside of the big toe can open the constricted blood vessels in the neck that are causing the migraine response. If you find that the pain of your migraine is most intense in the back of your head, try massaging the underside of the middle toe for additional pain relief.

Relaxation Techniques

Relaxation techniques are valuable tools to the migraine sufferer. Because stress is such a common trigger, if you can learn how to manage your stress response without medication, you can gain the upper hand in managing your pain. Any relaxation techniques are appropriate therapies for reducing the pain of migraine headaches. In addition to trying the few specific suggestions that follow, be sure to read the detailed explanations of each in Chapter 3.

Guided Visual Imagery

Guided visual imagery has proven especially effective in controlling the pain accompanying the migraine headache. It is most useful if you use guided imagery in the beginning stages of your headache, but even in the midst of the most painful attacks, patients have been able to take their mental focus away from the pain through this technique. To use guided imagery, close your eyes and compare your pain to a physical event. For example, you may see your migraine as a raging forest fire. View this scene in your mind and feel the pain it brings. Next, bring the scenario to a happy ending. Picture this forest fire being drowned by torrential rain. Tell yourself that as the fire goes out in your scene, so does your pain.

The number of imaginary scenes like this one that can be used to mentally "drown" your pain is limitless. Try making up several and then plan to use them when you have a migraine. After a while you'll get an idea of which ones work best for you.

Autogenic Training

This relaxation technique is actually a combination of guided imagery, meditation, and biofeedback. The ultimate goal is to regulate the body's blood flow and bring it back to a normalized rate. Because migraines are triggered by irregular blood flow, improved circulation will lessen the pain. Practicing autogenic training on a routine schedule can serve to reduce the frequency of migraine attacks.

Try this example of an autogenic exercise for migraine headaches:

Lie down in a comfortable position. Close your eyes and attempt to shut out all other thoughts, especially those of your headache. Since autogenics relies on getting a message to your unconscious mind, it is extremely important to concentrate on clearing the lines of communication to your unconscious mind. Next recite the following six lines over and over in a slightly audible tone:

1. My arms and legs are heavy.
2. My arms and legs are warm.
3. My heartbeat is calm and regular.
4. My breathing is calm and regular.
5. My abdomen is warm.
6. My forehead is cool.

With enough practice, soon you will be able to feel the results of this relaxation technique. By reciting these lines repeatedly, you can redirect the blood flow away from your forehead because you have convinced your mind that your forehead is "cool" and requires only a normalized flow of blood. This change in circulation can reduce the pain of a migraine.

Deep Breathing

Many times the pain of a migraine headache can be magnified by improper breathing, most specifically hyperventilation. When we are in danger, in a panic, or very anxious (as we might be when we sense a migraine is coming), we tend to take short, shallow breaths that reduce the amount of oxygen we take into our body. When you feel your migraine coming on, it's very possible that you exacerbate the pain by changing your breathing pattern. Deep-breathing exercises can help you normalize your breathing, which will reduce the intensity of your pain.

For prompt first aid for a bout of hyperventilation, breathe into a paper bag for about thirty seconds, rest, and then repeat the procedure until you feel more relaxed and your breathing pattern has returned to normal. Throughout the entire migraine period, monitor your breathing and try to keep your breaths deep and rhythmic.

Meditation

Any form of meditation, whether it is yoga or simply taking a quiet moment to yourself, will help you take your mind off your pain, thus changing the way you experience it. In the case of a migraine headache, meditation combined with deep breathing or guided imagery has proven especially helpful.

If your migraines occur quite frequently, it would be worthwhile to learn a disciplined type of meditation, such as yoga, that would consistently calm your body and mind and ward off the migraine stress response.

Biofeedback

Many studies have supported the use of biofeedback to reduce both the frequency and severity of migraine headaches. Biofeedback is one of the few natural therapies that is endorsed by the National Headache Foundation as a viable option to prescription drugs. In fact, biofeedback often is used to wean patients from their dependence on drugs to natural and holistic forms of medicine.

The main objective in a biofeedback session for the treatment of migraine is to increase the blood flow to the hands. When blood is directed to the hands, it reduces the rush of blood that has strained the vessels in and around the head area. As these blood vessels become less swollen, the head pain subsides.

You'll need professional help to learn the skill of biofeedback. But once you've learned how to control your response to your tension and migraines, you'll be able to practice this relaxation technique at home.

Migraine headaches cause such intense pain that it is quite understandable why you might beg your physician for some quick pill-popping remedy. Although many natural remedies also can be employed during a migraine attack to ease the pain, they generally do not offer such immediate relief and therefore may not meet your momentary need. The secret to managing the pain of migraine with natural remedies, therefore, is in prevention. If you can keep your body and mind healthy, balance the flow of your body energy, find and avoid your migraine triggers, and learn to manage your stress, you will soon find that you have reduced the frequency and intensity of your own headaches.

Chapter Seven

Temporomandibular Joint Dysfunction (TMJ)

To the millions of Americans who suffer temporomandibular joint dysfunction, the letters TMJ are more than just an acronym for what ails them—they are a code word for frustration and chronic pain.

Originally the name TMJ was given to pain or discomfort involving the movement or position of the mandible (jawbone). TMJ now is used to describe a wide array of ailments emanating from the head, neck, and jaw area, making the disorder difficult to diagnose. While the medical world debates what exactly constitutes TMJ, the exact number of sufferers remains equally elusive. Experts agree that millions go undiagnosed, untreated, or improperly diagnosed for years.

The vague quality of its symptoms, coupled with the high cost of conventional medicine, often leaves a patient suffering from TMJ confused and still in pain even after seeing many specialists and undergoing costly tests.

Fortunately, the future for TMJ sufferers looks brighter. Natural medicine often is considered for TMJ sufferers and in many cases has provided excellent results. Various effective natural remedies are discussed in this chapter, but first we explore the physiological world of TMJ and the conventional methods of treatment.

DEFINING TMJ

TMJ refers to pain or discomfort in the head, neck, or jaw area that involves the movement or position of the mandible (jawbone). Symptoms for this ailment range from a clicking or popping sound when the mouth is opened widely, to severe headaches, dizziness, earaches, and even sore muscles and muscle spasms in the neck and shoulder. Some 70 to 90 percent of TMJ patients indicate pain in jaw movement; 40 to 60 percent indicate unilateral joint noise; and 15 to 25 percent have a limited range of jaw motion.

For reasons unknown to modern science, nearly three-fourths of those suffering from TMJ are women; it should be noted, however, that recent studies suggest that the disorder may occur equally in both sexes but that women are more likely to seek treatment. Older research reported that most sufferers were women in their forties and fifties, but today's studies show an increasing number of men and women under the age of twenty who have TMJ symptoms.

Causative Factors

There are three possible causative factors in any TMJ dysfunction. With each patient these factors vary in importance and degree, but, generally speaking, all can play a role in producing the numerous symptoms of this disorder. These factors are:

1. Pathological mechanical stresses in the biting relationship (malocclusion)

2. Habit patterns—repetitive movements and positions of the lower jaw outside the range of normal functional positions (nail biting, excessive gum-chewing, grinding of the teeth, and so on)

3. Emotional stress—associated either with deep-rooted, long-term problems, or with problems having to do with daily concerns such as interpersonal relations or financial matters

Pathological mechanical stresses in the biting relationship or poor tooth alignment in either a closing position or a side-to-side movement of the lower jaw can contribute to the onset of TMJ. Mechanical stresses can be caused by one of several occurrences: a tooth loss, with subsequent shifting of adjacent teeth; a bridge placement; or a filling that does not conform to existing function.

Unusual habits concerning jaw movements also can cause TMJ. Habits such as teeth clenching, nail biting, lip and cheek biting, grinding of the teeth, placement of foreign objects such as pipes and pens between the teeth, and chewing on ice are all classified as habit patterns leading to TMJ. (Nearly 60 percent of TMJ patients habitually grind or clench their teeth, most without knowing it.) Although the degree of the effect of such habits depends on the frequency and intensity of the practice, in some cases hundreds of pounds of pressure per square inch are applied. This excessive force leads to the wearing down of teeth, loss of enamel, loosening of teeth, and, of course, TMJ and pain.

Stress alone is powerful enough to cause all the common TMJ symptoms even without accompanying bad habit patterns or malocclusions. When stress is present, bad oral habits may actually be the effect rather than the cause of TMJ. Stress can trigger nervous habits such as those just listed, and eventually these habits can lead to TMJ. Stress-related clenching and grinding, for example, is found in 70 to 80 percent of TMJ patients who experience muscle spasms.

MYOFASCIAL PAIN DYSFUNCTION

Myofascial pain dysfunction (MPD) is a disorder often confused with TMJ. MPD is the name given to pain or discomfort caused by inflammation of the tissue (called fascia) that surrounds many muscles in the head, neck, and jaw area. Other symptoms of MPD include one-sided general pain and pain or discomfort in a larger area of the head, including the temples, neck, and upper back and shoulders. Although similar to TMJ, when no obvious joint damage is present, the condition is diagnosed as MPD.

Like TMJ, MPD often is difficult to diagnose. In many cases, TMJ and MPD are mistaken for muscle contractions and migraine headaches. Also, sometimes diagnosis is difficult because a patient may have both MPD and TMJ at once. Because of the similarity of these dysfunctions, as well as the difficulty in pinpointing each, some doctors have begun to combine these dysfunctions under the broad title of temporomandibular disorders.

CONVENTIONAL MEDICINE FOR TMJ

Because TMJ sufferers experience pain or discomfort in a variety of areas including the teeth, facial or neck muscles, or the jaw, they often visit a host of clinicians. Dentists, neurologists, and orthopedists are only a few of the physicians who may face a patient complaining of pain in the head-neck-jaw area. Although most specialists are trained to identify and treat TMJ, dentists most commonly apply treatment.

During your initial physical evaluation, your physician or dentist will begin by asking about clicking and popping sounds as well as soreness. Next you will be tested for out-of-balance facial features. When facial muscles are placed under stress, they can cause a person to have uneven earlobes or perhaps one eye will appear to be higher than the other. Finally, the dentist or physician may use ultrasound to "hear" electrical impulses traveling through the jaw muscles that indicate whether the muscles are under strain.

Once a diagnosis of TMJ is established, the physician has a variety of treatment procedures to choose from.

Drug Therapy

Painkillers commonly are used to manage the pain of TMJ. Anti-inflammatory drugs, analgesics, and muscle relaxants, or any combination of the three, may be prescribed. If symptoms persist or if the patient shows signs of stress or anxiety, some practitioners will add a muscle relaxant such as Valium or Flexeril to this pharmacological plan.

Because TMJ is considered a chronic pain condition, drug therapy should be considered a potentially dangerous treatment approach. The negative side effects of long-term drug use, as detailed in Chapter 1, may be far too physically and mentally disruptive to be used for anything other than temporary relief of acute pain.

Surgery

Surgery is an appropriate treatment approach for only about 10 percent of TMJ dysfunction cases. In these rare situations, the patient has a temporomandibular joint so deformed or damaged that more conservative approaches can't be considered.

In the past, surgery for TMJ lasted, at times, as long as three hours and caused unsightly scars. In addition, patients who underwent these operations often faced the risk of facial paralysis. Most of the procedures used today are modifications and improvements on different types of surgeries performed in the past. Surgery today may include repositioning and repair of displaced disks, recontouring of articular bone, or diskectomy with implants. Many surgeries are performed using arthroscopic methods. Similar to the surgery used to repair the damaged knees of athletes, arthroscopy is performed by making two tiny incisions in front of the ear of the TMJ patient. An extremely thin fiberoptic device is inserted into the actual joint. This device takes a video image of the joint and relays it to a TV screen so the surgeon can see exactly what is wrong and how to fix it without cutting the area wide open.

Postoperative care is fairly standard in TMJ surgery. The patient's head is elevated to reduce edema while the physician looks for the standard signs of infection such as fever or redness and swelling. Antiemetics usually are prescribed since postoperative vomiting may irritate the area. Antibiotics, steroids, and analgesics are commonly prescribed postoperatively. A pressure dressing is applied that covers the patient's ears and is removed the day after surgery. The 2.5- to 3.0-centimeter incision is then left uncovered. Healing takes about six months; during that time the patient may continue to wear a bite plate and practice jaw exercises designed to improve jaw mobility.

Most TMJ patients should never see a hospital operating room or experience surgery in a doctor's office. If your physician recommends surgery as a first-step approach, find another doctor for a second opinion.

Dental Therapies

Although the majority of TMJ sufferers do not need surgery, many may need an oral appliance or some conservative occlusal grinding to relieve the pain.

Oral Appliances

The oral appliances most often used in the treatment of TMJ are the bite plate or night guard. These devices can be inserted and removed with ease. They work by separating the biting surfaces of the teeth by placing a flat plate between them. The plate frees the jaw from incorrect placement in the tooth cusps; it allows the jaw to slide freely; it prevents further damaging wear of the teeth; it slows the recession of the gums; and it allows the chewing muscles to work without resistance. The bite plate is worn during the day and is removed for meals.

Night guards are worn only at night, but serve the same purpose. They also prevent the damaging effects of nocturnal clenching and teeth grinding.

Occlusal Adjustment

Occlusal adjustment is a procedure that involves the grinding of teeth and bone to correct the position of the jaw. It is used for TMJ patients who make a clicking sound when opening and/or closing the mouth, have minimal pain, and show evidence of disk derangement.

The dental community is not in agreement on the advisability of using occlusal adjustment in the treatment of TMJ. If your dentist suggests this approach, you should get a second opinion and remember: Occlusal adjustment is an irreversible treatment. It should be used only after all other reasonable and reversible techniques have been tried without success.

Many physicians and dentists cling to the use of drugs, surgery, or other invasive treatments for TMJ. But fortunately, as the line between conventional and natural medicine begins to blur, many other physicians and dentists are turning to alternative therapies.

NATURAL MEDICINE FOR
THE TREATMENT OF TMJ

Acupuncture

Acupuncture is an effective remedy for the pain of TMJ. It can be administered to obtain symptomatic relief of the pain and also to redirect the obstructed energy flow that may be causing the problem. In addition, acupuncture can help decrease your experience of stress to help resolve the physical tension associated with TMJ.

Acupressure

Acupressure is an excellent way to eliminate TMJ pain. If you'd like to self-administer acupressure, you might try applying firm pressure for one minute to these potent points:

St 6: between the upper and lower jaw on the muscle that bulges when you clench your teeth together
SI 17: directly in front of your ear hole in the space that enlarges when you open your mouth
Lv 3: on top of your foot in the valley between the big toe and second toe
Li 4: in the webbing between the thumb and index finger at

the highest spot of the muscle when the thumb and index finger are brought close together (Use in combination with Lv 3 to relax the jaw.)

Botanical Medicine

Herbs can be used to relieve the pain of TMJ. Those having analgesic properties include *Salix alba* (white willow bark), passionflower, hops, and valerian. Check with an herbalist for the exact amount and form that can best treat your pain.

Chiropractic

Chiropractic medicine often is used as a treatment for TMJ. Because the temporomandibular joint is structurally involved in the cervical spine, adjustment of the vertebrae can be a highly effective treatment approach. If the cause of the TMJ pain is rooted in spinal alignment, chiropractic medicine can effect a complete cure. If the cause is related more specifically to a dental problem, then a spinal manipulation will offer only symptomatic relief.

Exercise

Therapy for TMJ includes a combination of various kinds of mobility, stretching, coordinating, and strengthening exercises. Active and passive stretching of specific muscles may be suggested along with passive range-of-motion techniques to improve joint mobility. To avoid further irritation or increased pain, these exercises need to be prescribed by a physician, dentist, or physical therapist. Once carefully explained and practiced with medical supervision, they can be used at home to strengthen the joint and ease the pain.

If the joint is too painful to be exercised, a physical therapist may use a vapocoolant spray to prepare the muscles. In this case, the patient is seated with nose, eyes, and ears covered with a towel. Then the therapist applies the spray, using a fine nozzle to the facial area at a distance of no less than eighteen inches. Following the path of the muscle fibers, the therapist will cover the area two to three times while the patient slowly opens and closes the mouth. The therapist then will begin massaging the muscle tissue in a passive manner in all directions—opening and closing the mouth, protruding and retruding the jaw, and moving it side to side. This procedure usually is repeated at the therapist's office every two to three days until the pain becomes more manageable.

Hydrotherapy

Hydrotherapy can be used to ease the pain of TMJ. Applying moist heat to the afflicted joint increases the blood flow and lessens the degree of muscle tension. A small towel heated with steam or a reusable hot pack is best when applied for fifteen minutes, three to four times a day.

Certain patients do not respond to heat alone; they find relief from contrast therapy. To apply this remedy, alternate five to eight minutes each of heat, then ice, then heat again.

Do not initially apply heat to pain caused by a direct blow to the jaw or temporomandibular joint. This acute pain requires ice therapy three to four times daily for ten to fifteen minutes for the first one to three days and, thereafter, heat alone on the same schedule for a week.

Hypnosis

Hypnosis has been used successfully in the treatment of TMJ. Hypnosis and self-hypnosis can be administered with the intent of reducing the amount of pain sensations experienced by the TMJ sufferers. Susceptible patients can be instructed, while under a trance, to feel no pain. This state of pain relief lasts for a time even after the hypnotic session.

A second use of hypnosis in the treatment of TMJ lies in its ability to help individuals break the oral habits that can cause or aggravate this ailment. While under hypnosis, for example, a patient may be "programmed" to stop teeth clenching or grinding. In this way the underlying cause of the problem is tackled at the same time the patient may be using other natural therapies to reduce the sensation of pain.

Nutrition

TMJ has many causative factors that can be treated effectively with nutritional therapy. If, for example, you experience headaches with this pain syndrome, this indicates a restriction of circulation and so you need to put more oxygen into your blood. You can do this by increasing your mineral intake and by adding exercise to your pain-management regimen. Both of these steps increase the oxygen content of the blood. Also, you can ask your doctor about taking a supplement called O^1 oxygen in homeopathic levels; this helps oxygen get into the cell, increasing circulation to the brain, thus getting rid of the TMJ symptoms.

The causative factors that contribute to TMJ are far too many to detail in this chapter, but whatever the cause, the nutritional approach remains very basically the same: You need to increase mineralization of the body; this will pull together all the waste matter that is stimulating the pain of TMJ.

Foods with high mineral content include all the root vegetables, such as beets, carrots, and sweet potatoes. You also can increase your mineral intake by taking food-based mineral supplements (supplements extracted from foods) such as dulse and kelp tablets. You should not take chemical-based mineral supplements; they actually can intensify the pain in the jaw.

However, if your case of TMJ is purely a structural problem (involving the placement of the jaw in the head), nutritional therapy cannot be used to treat the problem. However, a change of diet to soft foods may help ease the pain and discomfort. Although it's not necessary to restrict intake to gelatin and porridge, you should try to stay away from foods that put undue stress on the masticatory muscles of the jaw. Avoid foods difficult to chew such as meat, hard rolls, caramel, and nuts and stay away from foods that require wide jaw opening such as large rolls, pickles, or club sandwiches. As a temporary remedy, this will give the masticatory muscles a chance to rest and heal.

Psychotherapy

Because TMJ may be caused or aggravated by stress, a variety of psychological therapies can be used in its treatment.

Cognitive Therapy

It is now recognized that stress and tension are strongly influenced by personal appraisal and self-perception. How you perceive a particular stress in your life will have an effect on how that stress will affect your body. Cognitive therapy can help you think about life stresses in new ways; this readjustment of your thought processes can limit or eliminate tension responses that cause muscle tightness in the facial, head, and neck muscles and lead to teeth clenching and grinding—all of which cause or aggravate TMJ.

Cognitive therapy also can help you learn to think about the pain of TMJ in a different way. For one thing, positive thinking can raise your pain threshold. And second, giving yourself mental control over your pain reduces the feelings of helplessness that serve only to perpetuate pain.

Behavioral Therapy

Behavioral therapy is an appropriate approach to TMJ when oral habits are causative factors. This kind of therapy can help you break patterns such as biting nails; chewing gum or tobacco; clenching a pipe, cigar, or pens; and grinding or clenching teeth, which can be difficult (if not impossible) to eliminate without professional help.

A therapist also may help you ease the pain of TMJ by altering your sleep habits. To decrease pressure placed on the chewing muscles in the jaw area, you should sleep on a single flat pillow; this will place the cervical spine in a comfortable resting position. Also you should avoid resting on your stomach or side; these positions can stress the jaw and the temporomandibular joint.

An exception to this sleeping position is made in cases when a causative factor is teeth grinding. Sleeping on your side may put pressure on the nerves of the face that prompt grinding. If you now sleep on your side, try changing your position to your back. It usually takes three or four nights to adapt to this change of position. If you find the change difficult, you can ease the adjustment by propping pillows alongside your body to inhibit rolling.

If you find that you continually return to the side position during the night, you might try another approach: You can ease the pressure on the side of your face while sleeping on your side by sleeping on a soft pillow and by placing another pillow under your upper arm.

If you sleep with a spouse or companion, he or she can help break your habit of nocturnal grinding. Some studies have observed that teeth grinding (bruxism) takes place primarily during the fourth sleep stage of rapid eye movement (REM). Although there is no documented connection between dreams and grinding, some clinicians have helped teeth grinders reduce the frequency of their habit by repeatedly awakening them at the first signs of clenching or grinding. This method requires diligent attention, but the results after even one week may be significant enough to encourage you to continue until the habit is completely broken.

The process goes like this: The moment your sleep companion hears you begin to grind, he or she should wake you and have you relax your jaw completely; then reposition yourself on your back. Continue this procedure throughout the night every night for two weeks to see if it has a positive effect.

Other kinds of psychotherapy including couples, family, supportive, exploratory, psychoanalysis, and Gestalt also may be helpful in breaking the stress/pain connection that can cause TMJ. Psychotherapy is especially helpful when the cause of the stress is so deep rooted that the patients themselves aren't yet aware of what is causing their muscle strain and accompanying TMJ.

Relaxation Techniques

Relaxation techniques are very helpful in managing the pain of TMJ caused by emotional stress. The stress itself is not harmful, but stress tends to make us tense our facial muscles and tighten our jaws, promoting clenching, grinding, or gritting the teeth—and that causes pain.

The following relaxation techniques all have been used successfully to break these stress habits. They can even help stop nocturnal habits for these two reasons: When practiced immediately before bedtime, they reduce the jaw tension that builds up during the day and often seeks relief during sleep, and when practiced in the daytime, they retrain the body's stress response and again reduce jaw tension and overall stress buildup. You may have to experiment with each until you find the tactic or combination of tactics that gives you relief.

Guided Imagery

Guided imagery is a handy technique that can stop a stress response dead in its tracks. When you feel your jaw, mouth, or neck muscles tensing during a stressful moment, follow the guidelines suggested in Chapter 3 and imagine a relaxing, peaceful place where there is no tension or stress, where problems are banished, where you are safe and secure and comfortable. This mental image will help keep your muscles calm.

Deep Breathing

The deep-breathing exercises for TMJ pain follow the guidelines detailed in Chapter 3, but add an additional tactic to prevent the jaw from tensing. To ease the tension caused by stress, breathe in deeply and slowly *through a slightly opened mouth*. The open mouth keeps the jaw relaxed. These deep breaths interrupt the shallow breathing pattern that accompanies a stress response and bring in extra oxygen needed to fight off anxiety.

Muscle Relaxation

Progressive muscle relaxation is an effective weapon against stress. To target TMJ pain specifically, try this:

- Clench your teeth firmly for about five seconds.
- Relax for five seconds.
- Repeat this sequence four to six times a day.

Studies have found that as many as 75 percent of people who grind their teeth stop grinding after twenty-one days of this self-treatment. The key is consistency. If you try this approach, don't skip any exercise periods.

Any relaxation technique that calms your stress response will be effective in reducing the pain of stress-related TMJ. Tactics such as autogenic training, meditation, distraction, music, and laughter are all appropriate in this case.

Biofeedback

Biofeedback has proven to be effective in helping 60 to 70 percent of patients break the damaging oral habits that lead to TMJ dysfunction. Using electromyographic (EMG) biofeedback (at a cost equivalent to that of physical therapy), the patient gains control of neuromuscular structures. When the brain instructs groups of muscles (in this case, the muscles of the jaw, neck, or upper shoulder) to contract or stop contracting, small amounts of electrical energy are released. Biofeedback machines can detect and display this energy, helping the patient become more aware of this activity and how it can be controlled consciously.

Some patients improve after three to four sessions; others need one to three months of therapy. For those on longer-term treatment, some therapists suggest renting or buying equipment to use at home.

TENS

Most therapists reserve transcutaneous electrical nerve stimulation (TENS) for treating acute, intractable pain or for use in the office as a preliminary treatment for patients who are too sensitive to tolerate physical stretching and exercising. Among those who do use TENS, between 16 and 40 percent have partial to full relief of pain.

Some patients respond to only one session lasting thirty-five to forty minutes, while others will need several hours of stimulation. Once a physical therapist has helped you find the best site for the electrode and the most effective frequency, charge, and pulse rate, you can rent your own small stimulator for use at home.

Natural medicine is now becoming the preferred mode of treatment for TMJ among many physicians and dentists. Highlighting the preference for noninvasive techniques, the American Dental Association drafted the following guidelines in June 1992 for TMJ treatment:

• There is insufficient data comparing the different forms of therapy to establish a priority for their use, but conservative, reversible therapy is preferred when possible.

- A warm, positive, and reassuring attitude on the part of the clinician is crucial in the treatment of temporomandibular disorders.

- Short-term use of pharmacologic agents can be helpful. Therapy commonly includes use of nonaddictive analgesics, anti-inflammatory drugs, antianxiety agents, and muscle relaxants. Use of antidepressants is indicated less frequently.

- Consider occlusal adjustment therapy permanent. It is not indicated as a routine therapy.

- Occlusal appliances are recommended for many dysfunctions involving the chewing muscles and the temporomandibular joint, if they do not permanently reposition the teeth or jaw.

- Behavior therapies—biofeedback and other relaxation techniques—are indicated for dysfunction involving the chewing muscles.

- Consider surgery only after failure of currently acceptable nonsurgical treatments and based on a definitive diagnosis of pathologic joint disorder or anatomic defect.

- Meniscectomy, or surgery to remove the meniscus (articular disk), is indicated only when the meniscus is so deranged, damaged, or diseased that no alternative exists.

These guidelines further highlight the importance of first using conservative, noninvasive remedies in the treatment of TMJ.

CHAPTER EIGHT

Neurogenic Pain

Neurogenic pain is an excruciating, shooting pain that extends along the course of one or more nerve paths. It is usually described as being sharp, sudden, and intermittent. Almost any infection or disease that damages the peripheral nerves (those outside the spinal cord) may cause some form of neurogenic pain, which sometimes can be worse than the pain of the original problem. The variety of neurogenic conditions makes it difficult to generalize information about this pain syndrome, so this chapter looks at only a few of the most common. Although most of this chapter is pertinent to all kinds of neurogenic pain, check with your physician or therapist before beginning the suggested remedies.

First we take a brief overview of occipital, brachial, intercostal, and lumbar neuralgias; then we take a more in-depth look at the three most common neuralgias: postherpetic, trigeminal, and a related ailment, reflex sympathetic dystrophy.

NEURALGIAS

Occipital neuralgia causes pain in the back of the head from the hairline on the neck up to the area behind the ears. In some cases, merely touching the ends of the hair can produce severe pain.

Brachial neuralgia develops as a result of strained physical exercise, or exposure to severe cold, or from accumulation of fatigue after heavy labor. In many cases, severe pain persists even during times of rest.

Intercostal neuralgia produces severe pain in the chest region. Most often the pain shoots mainly from the left side of the back to the area below the nipple. The pain characteristically runs along the region of the ribs. It's often difficult to distinguish this problem from angina and pleurisy.

Lumbar neuralgia produces pain in the area of the lower back to the lower abdomen. It is commonly called lumbago, and the pain is often especially severe in the genital area. There are many varied causes of lumbar neuralgia. The most frequent and severe case is called cricked back, which develops into a vertebral hernia.

POSTHERPETIC NEURALGIA

Postherpetic neuralgia is caused by the herpes zoster virus, an acute viral infection characterized by nerve inflammation and skin eruptions. Also called shingles, this virus causes pain that usually subsides as the disease runs its course. But in some cases when the nerves have been affected, the pain can last for years.

The pain caused by this neuralgia often is aggravated by almost any type of stimulus. Things such as external noises or covering the affected area with clothing have been known to intensify the pain. Stress and emotional upset too may exacerbate the pain of postherpetic neuralgia.

TRIGEMINAL NEURALGIA

Trigeminal neuralgia (or tic douloureux) is a condition affecting the nerves of the face. Its general characteristics are these:

- It occurs mostly in older people.
- It most commonly affects the right side of the face.
- It is found in women more often than in men, although why this difference exists is not clearly understood.
- The pain can occur spontaneously, but in most cases it is triggered by a variety of stimuli such as eating, talking, washing, brushing teeth, shaving, or exposure to cold winds.

The pain associated with this neuralgia is thought to be caused by pressure exerted by a blood vessel pulsating against the junction of the central and peripheral myelin layers (the protective coating enveloping all of the body's nerves) of the trigeminal nerve next to the brain stem. In 80 percent of cases, arteries cause the pressure on the nerves. Veins have been cited as the culprit in approximately 8 percent of cases, tumors in 5 to 8 percent, and multiple sclerosis in 2 to 3 percent. Other causes of trigeminal neuralgia include aneurysms and angiomas. In some cases no cause at all is found.

Patients describe the pain of trigeminal neuralgia as a piercing, knifelike sensation. During the few seconds or minutes that the pain lasts, the patient is stunned and unable to speak. A pain-free period lasting from a few hours to a few days follows the attack, and total remission does occur, which, depending on the patient, may last from a month or two to several years.

REFLEX SYMPATHETIC DYSTROPHY
(RDS)

Although not classified as a medical neuralgia, reflex sympathetic dystrophy (also known as RDS, causalgia, and Sudeck's atrophy) does share common properties with other neuralgias and is often grouped with neurogenic disorders.

RSD is an extremely painful condition. It is usually the result of a trauma such as a crash injury, fracture, or sprain. Its symptoms are burning pain, vasoconstriction, skin changes, coldness of the affected limb, and limited movement.

A physician will diagnose the patient based on a physical examination and evaluation by thermography and three-stage bone scan. Treatment is given according to the stage of the patient's condition. The four stages are:

1. Characteristic pain and sweating; coldness in the affected area
2. An extension of stage 1 and a limited range of movement
3. A significant restriction of range of movement and symptoms caused by lack of adequate nutrition to the tissues via the blood supply
4. Presence of a frozen and useless extremity

Early diagnosis is crucial because successful treatment depends on early intervention.

CONVENTIONAL TREATMENT
OF NEURALGIAS

Drug Therapy

Neuralgias often are treated with a combination of medications. Antidepressants, anticonvulsants, and major tranquilizers commonly are prescribed to ease the pain. Unfortunately, the negative side effects of these drugs include drowsiness, dizziness, nausea, dry mouth, and even aplastic anemia along with tolerance and addiction. For these reasons, drug therapy may not be an appropriate long-term treatment for the pain of neuralgia.

Local injections of a steroid or anesthetic are used sometimes to control the pain of this condition. Although effective, this approach should not be considered a long-term cure. The relief lasts only as long or slightly longer than the effects of the drug. If you're an outpatient, this can mean returning to your physician for an injection every day. Also, trigger-point injections treat only the symptom of pain and not the cause, so the pain will always return. In addition, because injections can aggravate the condition, often the pain returns with more intensity than before. And finally, the body can develop a tolerance for the drug and require more frequent injections with reduced effect.

Surgery

Surgery sometimes is performed in an attempt to stop the pain of a neuralgia. The most commonly used procedures involve cutting the affected nerves or heating them until the fibers are destroyed. Unfortunately, the side effects of surgical treatment can be profound; the approach should be used only as a last resort and always with great caution.

Cutting or heating the nerves carrying the pain signal can cause a total loss of sensation and permanent numbness in the affected area. Also, surgery doesn't guarantee that the pain will be eliminated because nerves have the resilient capacity to regenerate themselves. Indeed, when neurogenic pain returns after surgical treatment, the pain can be more intense than it was before surgery.

Less invasive surgical procedures that seem to cause fewer side effects are being introduced in some cases. A dorsal column stimulator can be surgically implanted into the spine at the area affected by pain. This device acts like an internal TENS unit that can be self-regulated. It has been found to manage some kinds of neurogenic pain effectively. Also, internal infusion pumps sometimes are recommended. In a surgical procedure, a catheter is inserted into the epidural space (between the spinal cord and the vertebrae) and a small thermosensitive pump is implanted in the patient's side. Continuous morphine or an anesthetic is pumped into the epidural space. Relatively speaking, the surgical aspect of this procedure is without negative side effects, but the continuous infusion of drugs carries with it the negative consequences of any long-term drug therapy.

Traditional medicine has a limited store of treatment approaches for the pain of neuralgia. It is a persistent and complex condition generally unresponsive to drugs or surgery in the long run. Fortunately, alternative medicine offers you a variety of ways to treat this pain effectively and naturally without negative side effects.

NATURAL MEDICINE FOR
NEUROGENIC PAIN

Acupuncture

Acupuncture often is remarkably effective in treating neurogenic pain, especially when treatment is begun close to the onset of the pain and before it becomes chronic. However, even chronic pain can be diminished through appropriate treatment.

Usually a course of twelve treatments will give you a sense of the effectiveness of the modality. Treatment will vary depending on the location of the pain as well as its quality. Your acupuncturist will have to do a careful Oriental medical diagnosis. There is not just one cause of neuralgias in Chinese medicine, and two people presenting with the same Western diagnosis may have quite different Oriental medical diagnoses.

If your case is more severe, you may need to combine acupuncture with other natural modalities such as chiropractic treatment for complete relief. In some advanced cases, a cure through acupuncture may not be possible, but still this therapy can be used effectively to manage your pain.

Botanical Medicine

Although often thought of as a spice, horseradish has long been revered for its healing powers. Externally, fresh chopped or grated horseradish can be mixed with a little water and applied as a heat-producing and pain-relieving compress for any type of neuralgia.

In addition, pain relief can be found in *Salix alba* (white willow bark), passionflower, hops, and valerian. Consult a qualified herbalist about the remedy and amount appropriate for you.

Exercise

As a form of relaxation and a means of increasing the body's oxygen intake (which increases the absorption of nutrients), exercise often is used as an adjunct therapy in the treatment of neurogenic pain.

Also, in some cases exercise prescribed by a physical therapist can reduce neurogenic pain. For patients with RDS, it increase the chances of regaining use of the affected limb.

Hydrotherapy

Hydrotherapy can be used effectively to ease the symptomatic pain of various neuralgias. Although it is not an effective long-term therapy, hot and cold applications can offer some relief and can be incorporated into a natural medicine pain-relief program. Ask your physician for the kind of application that is most appropriate to your particular kind of neuralgia.

Hypnosis

Hypnosis can be used successfully to treat neurogenic pain. For the most part, hypnosis is a recommended therapy for pain that is exacerbated by stress, tension, or anxiety. Although most types of neurogenic pain have a specific organic root, some patients have noticed a connection between the degree of pain they feel and the tension in their life at the moment. If your neuralgia seems to be aggravated by stress and is responsive to relaxation therapies, it may well be treated through hypnosis.

Nutrition

Because the sensation of pain is caused by the nervous system's reaction to the level of acidity in the body, and neurogenic pain emanates from the nerve pathways, nutritional therapy is a most effective approach to the treatment of neuralgias. A high acidity level in the body is an aggravant that will constantly irritate the pain condition. The primary objective of nutritional therapy for neuralgia, then, is to alkalinize the body.

Alkalinization can be achieved by a definitive change in diet. You should eliminate pollutants such as coffee, cigarettes, and alcohol. You also must reduce your intake of acid-based foods such as meats, cheese, white breads, and processed foods. Replace these foods with those having a high pH level such as vegetables, fruits, grains, and beans, along with alkaline vegetable juices such as homemade celery or cucumber juice.

When you achieve total alkalinization of the bloodstream, you will reduce your pain. Continued attention to your alkalinized diet will help soothe your neurogenic pain condition.

Psychotherapy

Cognitive Therapy

Cognitive therapy is a useful psychological treatment for neurogenic pain when used in conjunction with other pain-relief methods. Cognitive therapy can help you think differ-

ently about your pain as well as relieve some of the distress
and anxiety associated with it. It can help you recognize the
kinds of thoughts and bodily responses you have to your
pain. It can teach you to focus your attention in ways that
will ease the intensity of the pain and in some cases even
abort an attack.

Behavioral Therapy

Behavioral therapy can help you recognize and change
the pain behaviors you may have adopted in response to
your pain. Actions such as excessive bed rest, moaning,
complaining, and social isolation can become habitual and
in fact may be aggravating and sustaining the pain.

Couples and Family Therapy

Because your pain also affects those around you, marital
and family therapy may be a beneficial component of your
pain-management program. Family members also need to
learn all about your ailment and understand the psychological toll chronic pain can take on relationships. In therapy,
family members will learn how they may unknowingly be
contributing to the cycle of chronic pain by supporting your
pain behaviors when they do things such as take over your
tasks or encourage bed rest and a passive response to the
pain.

Relaxation Techniques

Neurogenic pain can be aggravated or even instigated by
stress. When you're upset, angry, anxious, or depressed,
your muscles tense, your breathing becomes shallow and
faster, and the blood flow throughout your body is re-

stricted. All of these physical stress reactions affect your nervous system and therefore can influence your pain experience. Learning to calm the stress response can help you manage your condition. The following relaxation exercises are suggested natural remedies for neurogenic pain; be sure also to read the full discussion of relaxation and its effect on pain on pages 91–107.

Guided Imagery and Meditation

This relaxation therapy is a useful technique because you can do it in many settings.

One type of meditation proven especially helpful uses guided imagery to create movies of the mind. These are short ad-libbed meditations that can reduce pain temporarily. The technique helps you visualize your nerve pathways as healthy and nonpainful in an attempt to "trick" your brain into producing sensations of calm and comfort.

As you feel the pain begin, for example, you might say to yourself:

> *The nerve pathway is not inflamed. It is healthy and strong. I feel no pain. The muscles around these nerves are relaxed and smooth. I can feel and see rich red blood flow through this area bringing oxygen and nutrients that keep the pain away. I can see myself walking without pain. I see myself enjoying my life without pain.*

Autogenic Training

Autogenic training can be used to relieve the pain of neuralgia. It enables you to focus your attention on particular parts of your body without putting any physical pressure on your affected nerves.

Deep Breathing

Deep-breathing exercises can effectively stop the body's stress response. This gives you the ability to control the muscle tension that can trigger your pain.

Progressive Muscle Relaxation

Progressive muscle relaxation can be used to ease the pain of a neuralgia. However, it's best to avoid tensing muscles around the affected area because this can aggravate your condition.

Distraction

Although distraction techniques such as music, laughter, and socializing don't stop neurogenic pain, they do have a place in your pain-management program. When the mind is distracted by other stimuli, it is not able to process persistent pain signals as easily as when you're unoccupied. If you can resist the temptation to take to your bed when your pain begins, you'll find yourself experiencing less discomfort.

Biofeedback

Biofeedback can help some neuralgia patients control their response to pain. If you find that your pain episodes are worsened by stress, investigating the benefits of this technique certainly would be worthwhile. Learning to control your blood pressure and body temperature voluntarily gives you a great sense of control over your health and well-being.

CHAPTER NINE

Terminal Cancer

An estimated one in four Americans will have cancer at some time. Although many battle this common enemy, each person has a unique experience with the pain of the disease. Many types of cancer are curable, and their pain lasts for a limited "acute" period of time. Other kinds of cancer are not painful at all, even in the final stages. But in 87 percent of terminal cancer cases, pain is the debilitating companion of this progressive malignant disease. It is these painful terminal cancers that are the subject of this chapter.

As a terminal cancer patient, you certainly have many things to think about—most likely personal, social, medical, and financial worries crowd your day for attention. But, despite all these concerns, you can't lose sight of the fact that you are alive *today* and you don't have to accept intolerable pain as your constant companion. There are things you can do to make your life less painful, letting you concentrate on the pleasurable things that are really important to you now.

In some ways cancer pain is similar to other kinds of pain. It is like acute pain in its continuous release of urgent signals, in its management with narcotic analgesics, and in its treatment directed toward the underlying disease. It's also much like chronic pain in its persistence and accompanying chronic distress and disability, which gives it many of the psychological components of chronic pain. But the pain caused by the growth of an untreatable malignant tumor is considered to be a progressive or unmanageable pain that is in a category of its own.

CAUSES OF CANCER PAIN

There are three kinds of cancer pain syndromes: pain due to the progression of the disease, pain caused by the treatment therapies, and pain unrelated to the cancer itself.

If you have cancer, you'll need to distinguish the root of your pain in order to supplement your medical treatment with natural therapies most successfully.

Pain Due to the Progression of the Disease

In a report prepared for Roche Laboratories in 1981, K. M. Foley reported that 78 percent of cancer pain is due to the progression of the disease. Reasons for the pain include the following:

• Sometimes a tumor puts direct pressure on surrounding nerves. This often causes a continuous, sharp, boring-type pain. It may be mild in the early stages, later becoming more severe depending on the growth rate of the tumor and the nerve structures involved.

• Obstruction of blood vessels or lymphatics is a common cause of cancer pain. Blockage of an artery decreases blood supply and causes numbness, weakness, and deep-aching discomfort.

• Obstruction of veins causes swelling, engorgement, tightness, and fullness of the body part, with a bluish-red appearance.

• Another type of pain is produced when a cancer mass blocks a portion of the intestinal tract. This can cause distention of the abdomen and gripping continuous pain.

• Cancer often causes swelling and thickening in areas containing many pain-sensitive structures such as connective tissues or bone-covering tissues.

• Tumors in some body areas occasionally feel extremely painful if they cause tissue destruction, infection, and inflammation.

As the causes of pain differ, so too does the pain itself. As best as one can give words to the pain experience, the different types of cancer pain caused by the progression of the disease might be described in this way:

Bone tumors An expanding bone lesion will irritate and stretch the nerve-rich bone-covering tissue; this causes an intermittent, yet severe, continuous, dull, and deep, shooting or piercing pain that is difficult to tolerate. Bone tumors can originate in the bone or travel to the bone from another cancerous area. Breast and prostate cancer, for example, can metastasize to the vertebrae, to the bones of the arms and legs, or to the pain-sensitive portions of the brain and skull. Melanoma also may spread to all of these structures. Tumors of the kidney also occasionally spread to the bone.

Stomach Cancer Causes burning, ulcer-type pain.

Pancreas Causes vague aching in the upper-back region and pit of the stomach, with feelings of indigestion, excess stomach acidity, and burning.

Intestinal cancer   Causes gripping pain and bloating.

Lung cancer   Often involves the sensitive covering of the lungs (pleura) or the bones of the rib cage; it may also block air passages and blood vessels causing pneumonia.

Bladder   Causes fullness, burning, and irritation.

Uterus or uterine cervix   Causes pelvic pressure and bladder irritation in late states.

Cancers not frequently associated with pain are those of the larynx, esophagus, liver, lymphatic tissues, blood-forming tissues, muscles, and reproductive organs.

Pain Caused by Treatment Therapies

K. M. Foley found that 19 percent of cancer pain syndromes result from treatment therapies such as surgery, radiation, and chemotherapy. If you've had surgery, you may have experienced pain in the postoperative period and also may have developed incisional neuritis from cutting sensory fibers during surgery.

Radiation may result in fibrosis or even death of connective tissue and suppression of the immune system. It also can cause your skin to feel painful, and it can result in bowel changes.

If you have received chemotherapy, you may have developed secondary pain syndromes. For example, some chemotherapeutic agents cause painful nerve damage; others suppress the immune system, leaving the patient at high risk for various and painful infectious bacterial and viral illnesses. Chemotherapy also can cause a painful mouth irritation.

Pain Unrelated to the Cancer

Three percent of the pain problems experienced by cancer patients are unrelated to the disease itself. In addition to your cancer, you may suffer any of the acute or chronic pain syndromes found in the general population. These can include arthritis, diabetic neuropathy, myofascial pain syndromes, and others discussed in this book. Sometimes these conditions exist completely separate from the cancer pain. Other times, the patient's perception of and vulnerability to pain is heightened because of the cancer, and so the "unrelated" pain is indeed affected by the cancer pain and often will respond to cancer pain treatment.

CONVENTIONAL MEDICINE FOR CANCER PAIN

Conventional treatment of terminal cancer focuses on drug therapy, radiation and/or chemotherapy, and surgery. Since cancer pain is quite different from any other chronic pain, prudent use of conventional medicine is most often necessary, useful, and effective in treating this malignant disease. The combined effect of conventional and natural methods gives you a variety of ways to do something about your pain. Even cancer pain is not something that just has to be accepted. Indeed, all methods of pain management should be considered because pain itself actually can be harmful to the cancer patient's condition. Researchers Woodforde and Fielding have reported that in comparing cancer patients with and without pain, those with pain were significantly more emotionally disturbed, responded more poorly to treatment, and even died sooner.

This is only logical. We know that pain does not exist in a vacuum, but rather affects many other functions of the body and spirit. Pain can weaken the body's immune response, making it more susceptible to disease, and for the terminally ill cancer patient, additional disease and/or infection can cause life-threatening complications. Indeed, some studies have shown that the experience of pain may even suppress tumor-fighting cells. Pain management during drug therapy, radiation/chemotherapy, or surgery may bring you relief, thereby reducing the degree of social and psychological problems common in terminal illnesses, which could interfere with the positive effects of natural medicine as an adjunct therapy.

Drug Therapy

Drug therapy for terminal cancer pain runs the gamut from aspirin to morphine. In recent years it has become increasingly complex with the advent of multiple medications, adjunct drugs, and complex delivery systems such as patient-controlled analgesia (PCA) pumps, epidural catheters, and continuous parenteral infusions. But regardless of the drug or mode of delivery, the goal in all cases is to find medication that will ease the suffering with limited debilitating side effects.

Potent narcotic analgesics are the drug of choice in many cases. Unfortunately, they produce the most undesirable side effects. Common opiates such as morphine and methadone can cause drowsiness, lethargy, loss of interest in normally pleasant daily activities, decreased sexual interest, loss of appetite, weight loss, and constipation.

On the positive side of narcotic drug use, addiction is rarely a problem. According to a study published in *American Health* in November 1991, the effects of narcotics in recreational use is different from the effects found in therapeutic use. The researchers found that narcotics such as morphine do trigger euphoria in recreational users, but the overwhelming majority of cancer patients who get pain relief from morphine don't become addicted. Typically, as pain abates, these patients willingly accept lower dosages. Boston researchers who studied 11,882 hospital patients given opioids support this assertion. These researchers found that only four patients became drug abusers—and only one of them was a serious case. People living with the intractable pain of cancer find no euphoria from narcotic use—only relief.

Nerve blocks are another way of delivering drug therapy to cancer patients. Drug injections can act like a shot of Novocain before dental work, to stop the sensation of pain. Unfortunately, the relief is short-lived, requiring repeated injections, which is very inconvenient for outpatients. Also, because the injection can aggravate the condition, often the pain returns with more intensity than before. At the same time, the body develops a tolerance to the anesthesia, requiring more frequent injections with reduced effect.

Radiation/Chemotherapy

Radiation and chemotherapy (also called radiotherapy or irradiation therapy) can ease the pain of cancer as they kill or shrink cancer cells. Although effective, each treatment has negative side effects; you should discuss this with your physician to be sure the possible benefits will outweigh the negative side effects.

Surgery

Four different kinds of surgical procedures can reduce the pain of cancer: (1) removal or containment of the disease;

(2) relief of blockages caused by secondary problems such as intestinal obstruction; (3) removal of infected or dead body tissue; and (4) neurological surgery to intercept the pain message as it travels through the spine to the brain.

In any circumstance, treatment through surgery is a major undertaking with possibly serious side effects, and cancer surgery is no exception. For this reason, many professionals believe surgery should be a last resort after drug therapy, radiation and/or chemotherapy, and the implementation of natural remedies. And certainly—in the case of late-stage terminal cancer—it should be resorted to only after thoroughly weighing the pros and cons and the quality-of-life factor.

Drug therapy, radiation/chemotherapy, and surgery can all help to relieve cancer pain; in fact, recent medical and technological advances in all these areas of care have enabled many terminal patients to survive their disease for longer and longer periods of time. But as more people live with cancer, the emotional components of pain such as depression, fear, dependency, social isolation, and numerous pain behaviors need more attention. Natural therapies can help you better deal with the mind/body aspect of your cancer and further ease your pain.

NATURAL MEDICINE
FOR THE TREATMENT
OF CANCER PAIN

The most comprehensive pain-management program for terminal cancer combines conventional and natural remedies. Prudent use of medication, radiation/chemotherapy, and surgery can be much more effective when used along with the following natural therapies. Be sure to read Chapter 3 for a complete discussion of how each of these remedies works to ease chronic pain.

Acupuncture and Acupressure

Acupuncture and acupressure can be used with caution in the treatment of cancer pain. Both are especially helpful in relieving the physical distress caused by radiation and chemotherapy. And often these modes of Oriental medicine can effectively reduce the pain of cancer itself.

It is vital that the practitioner have training and experience in treating cancer. When this is the case, acupuncture can help the body's own healing defenses and mechanisms cope with, neutralize, and/or reverse the process of the cancer itself.

Botanical Medicine

If your physician has suggested that your pain may be managed with aspirin, you can trade in your aspirin bottle for an herb called *Salix alba*. Made from the white willow bark, this herb is the natural form of the salicylic found in aspirin.

Exercise

Too often bed rest is the recommendation for cancer pain. True, bed rest is necessary at times for some patients, but if you have the strength to walk, too much bed rest is harmful both physically and mentally.

Exercise can ease the pain of cancer in several ways:

- It can be used as relaxation, which can reduce the stress of the disease and the accompanying pain of tension.
- Exercise also can improve your strength and flexibility, giving you a sense of independence and health.
- Exercise can increase the level of the body's natural painkillers, endorphins.
- Exercise is a therapeutic approach to treating the constipation pain caused by some cancer treatments.

A particularly illustrative study on the use of exercise to treat cancer pain was reported in the *Clinical Pain Journal* in 1992. Researchers Terman and Loeser present the case of a sixty-two-year-old woman with cervical myelopathy and a diagnosis of a spinal cord tumor who was referred to the University of Washington Medical Center complaining of chest tightness, multiple joint pains, nausea, constipation, seizures, and deteriorating memory. At the time of admission she was confined to her bed with a full-time attendant and was receiving 240 milligrams of intravenous morphine per hour for her pain. This therapy gave her undesirable side effects and did not reduce her pain complaints or improve her functioning. Diagnostic studies failed to find any evidence of neoplasm and revealed only an old hemorrhage within the cervical spinal cord. A program of increasing physical and occupational therapy and decreasing opiate intake was initiated. Within one month, the patient's pain complaints decreased, as did the rest of her presenting complaints. Her activities of daily living greatly increased, making attendant care no longer necessary. In this case, physical movement had more healing and pain-relief power than even morphine.

It is impossible for us to prescribe a specific exercise program to relieve the pain specific to the many kinds of cancer. But be sure to ask your doctor or a pain-control specialist at a pain clinic for an exercise routine tailored to your needs and abilities. The benefits can be amazing.

Hydrotherapy

Hydrotherapy may be an appropriate way to relieve the discomfort of certain kinds of cancer pain, but first you must talk to your doctor about this therapy. The unsupervised use of hot or cold applications can, in some cases, be detrimental to your condition.

Hypnosis

In patients susceptible to the powers of hypnosis, this therapy can be used to help control the pain of terminal cancer along with the nausea, anxiety, and other unpleasant side effects of its treatment. One of many studies verifying this use of hypnosis was conducted in 1983 by researchers Spiegel and Bloom who investigated pain and mood disturbance of fifty-four women with metastatic breast cancer. The participants were randomly assigned to one of three groups: therapy group with self-hypnosis training emphasizing competence at mastering cancer-related pain and stress, therapy group without hypnosis, and a control group. At the end of the study, the self-hypnosis group demonstrated significantly less pain sensation and suffering.

If you have a positive attitude toward hypnosis and are motivated to give it a try, natural therapy may be able to give you self-controlled pain relief. A trained hypnotist (or even a self-help book) can teach you how to practice self-hypnosis anytime you need it—without cost, negative side effects, or the inconvenience of being dependent on a practitioner.

Nutrition

Cancer pain caused by the tumor itself pressing on tissue
and nerves cannot be remedied through nutritional therapy.

In other instances, cancer pain can occur when the cancer begins to "eat" at the body tissue, as happens with
breast cancer, for example. In these cases, natural nutrition
therapies in ointment form can be very effective in relieving cancer pain. On open wounds and visible skin irritations
like those found in melanomas, ointments including com-
frey packs, garlic packs, and chlorophyll can cause the cancer to go into remission. These ointments are especially
effective if at the same time you change your diet to eliminate pollutants such as caffeine, nicotine, and alcohol, and
you reduce body acidity by eliminating meats, cheese,
white breads, and processed foods and increase alkalinizing
foods such as vegetables, fruits, grains, and beans.

Psychotherapy

Psychotherapy can be an invaluable pain-control therapy.
In any form recommended by a mental health care provider or physician, therapy for the mind is an integral part
of natural medicine for cancer pain.

Cognitive-Behavioral Therapy

The way you think about cancer and the way you act on
those thoughts certainly does affect the degree, intensity,
and frequency of your pain. That's why cognitive and behavioral therapies are very helpful adjuncts to cancer treatments. Through cognitive therapy you can learn to replace
fearful and negative thoughts with courageous and con-

structive ones. Behavioral therapy can teach you how to monitor and reduce pain behaviors such as complaining, obsessing, excessive bed rest, social isolation, worrying, and the like that exacerbate pain. Indeed, a therapist can encourage a positive attitude and lifestyle that includes proper exercise, rest, diet, and socializing to actually give your immune system strength.

Family Therapy

Chronic cancer pain places an intense burden not only on you but on your entire family as well. Both you and your family must contend with family structure changes and tension and conflicts brought on by the disease, so family therapy is always a good idea in this circumstance.

One problem specific to terminal illness that can be addressed in family therapy is the alienation problem that occurs when family members begin the separation process too early. This emotional separation can deepen your feelings of hopelessness, helplessness, loneliness, and depression, increasing your perception of pain. Also, the family's method of expressing grief and anger can increase your own depression, anxiety, and grief. All of these very personal family communications can be addressed productively in family counseling sessions.

Family therapy also gives the family members a chance to talk about their feelings. By relieving their own emotional pain, they can deal more objectively with you. Sometimes your loved one takes a deep breath for the first time in a long time when a sympathetic therapist asks, "What's it like for *you* living with someone in constant pain?"

Supportive Therapy

Group therapy sessions are very beneficial in helping cancer patients deal with their pain. These meetings provide a place to share experiences, information about medical procedures, fears and concerns as well as hopes and triumphs. Here is a place where people won't shy away from you, or change the subject, or wince at the word "cancer."

Relaxation Techniques

Natural medicine plays an important role in the treatment of cancer pain by contributing to your emotional and psychological well-being. The pain of your cancer has a physical root, but still, the way you think about the pain and react to it will dramatically affect how you experience it. Stress, anxiety, tension, and fear are unavoidable companions of the cancer experience—all are also known to exacerbate pain. It is quite common, for example, for patients with uncontrolled cancer pain to develop conflicts with their family members and friends. Also, self-esteem is damaged because the cancer patient's appearance often deteriorates due to the progression of the disease, the cancer treatments, and the prolonged suffering. Many terminally ill cancer patients must quit their jobs, causing both economic hardship and an increase in feelings of dependency and uselessness. Quite clearly, therapies that can improve psychological functioning can help you better manage your pain.

Relaxation techniques including deep breathing, autogenic training, meditation, progressive muscle relaxation (with caution), and laughter all have been found to reduce cancer pain. See Chapter 3 for a complete discussion of these techniques and how they can have a positive effect on pain.

In addition and perhaps most notably, guided imagery, distraction, music, and biofeedback have been found to influence the perception of cancer pain.

Guided Imagery

Guided imagery is an effective technique for taking your mental focus off your pain. Building an imaginary place that is comfortable, carefree, and pain-free gives you a place in your mind where you can go when pain seems inescapable. Combined with meditation and/or deep-breathing techniques, this natural therapy can ease many of the stress-related pains of cancer.

Another kind of guided imagery called movies of the mind also is helpful in controlling cancer pain. Carl Simonton, M.D., and Stephanie Matthews-Simonton have pioneered the use of imagery techniques that often have significantly extended the life spans of hundreds of cancer patients. In addition to conventional therapy, the Simontons' techniques encourage patients to imagine scenes like this:

> *I can see my cancer. It is beginning to fall apart into pieces. It looks like shattered hamburger meat. Now I can see my white blood cells rushing to the scene. They are gobbling up the meat. They are devouring my cancer. White knights stand guard over the battle; they keep stray pieces from straying to other parts of my body.*

Try this kind of image several times every day. Really focus on the mental action. Advocates of the Simontons say it works!

Distraction

Fear and a sense of helplessness may keep you from social and functional activities. Yet avoiding pleasurable and purposeful events only contributes to the emotional agony of the disease and therefore can increase the feeling of pain. This is why a program of planned distraction can be a very helpful strategy. A walk, a car ride, a social or religious event, a visit with family and friends can all be used as modes of pain control. Without a doubt, if you withdraw from life, you'll feel more pain.

Music

As a relaxation and distraction technique, music has proven helpful in relieving cancer pain. One recent study out of the University of Nebraska Medical Center found that music, over a thirty-minute interval, is effective as an adjunct therapy in the reduction of cancer pain. This study was followed by a University of Utah study in which fifteen outpatients with cancer-related pain were assigned three days of twice-daily forty-five-minute sessions at home in which they listened to relaxing music. While the music was not found to affect mood significantly, eleven patients reported some reduction in pain and seven of those showed a moderate or great response. Try it!

Set aside a time twice a day to listen to your favorite kind of music. It can be anything from hard rock to classical violin—as long as you like it. Rest in a comfortable position and focus your thoughts on the music for about forty-five minutes. Chase away any other thoughts or mental disruptions and try to concentrate on the sounds you hear. After doing this for several days, you may find yourself looking forward to your pain-free music time.

Biofeedback

Biofeedback is a method of measuring how well one can use relaxation techniques to control the body's negative stress response. Because stress does contribute to the pain of cancer, biofeedback can be effective as a natural remedy. Ask your physician to refer you to a therapist who can teach you the secrets of biofeedback. In just a short time, you'll be able to lower your heart rate and blood pressure and raise your body temperature, all for the purpose of reducing your physical stress response that's been aggravating your pain.

TENS

Transcutaneous electrical nerve stimulation can be used to treat the pain of some kinds of cancer. Ask your physician if you are a candidate for this therapy. You will need a prescription and a fitting and then, with a turn of the dial, you may find pain relief.

Many medical experts believe that the fear of unmanageable pain is far greater than the fear of death. Sadly, you may face both of these concerns. It is our belief that in addition to conventional medicine's management of cancer, you need to know that you also can find pain relief and an improved quality of life in natural remedies.

CHAPTER TEN

Musculoskeletal Pain

When you slam that backhand shot across the tennis net, does your elbow cry out? When you wake in the morning, does your stiff neck remind you of your car accident a few years ago? When it rains, does the pain in your ankle bring back memories of an old sports injury? Do you think twice before picking up a heavy box for fear of "throwing out" your back again? All these chronic pain conditions can be grouped together and called musculoskeletal pain syndromes—pain caused by abnormal pressure of muscles and bones on adjacent nerves.

Your body is a complex system of bones that are bound together by ligaments and are moved, supported, and protected by muscles. These bones meet at joints that are enclosed in sleeves of tough, fibrous tissue that secrete a special lubricant called synovial fluid. The ends of your bones are protected by smooth yet tough cartilage. When all is working well, the musculoskeletal system is an amazing machine. But when this harmonious, efficient system is disrupted by vulnerable or injured bone sites and/or weak or injured muscles, the effect can be painful—very painful.

Some of the most common of these pain conditions have been discussed fully in their own chapters. Back pain, TMJ, some forms of arthritis, cancer pain, and pain in the elderly all involve the musculoskeletal system. There are also innumerable other musculoskeletal conditions that can't be addressed here individually but that surely cause chronic suffering and can be considered as a group in this chapter.

SKELETAL PAIN

There are three common causes of chronic skeletal pain: bone degeneration (as in osteoporosis), bone breakage or injury (as in a broken leg or vertebral whiplash), and congenital bone disorder (such as scoliosis). The pain of these bone conditions generally is localized to the affected area and is diagnosed easily.

Bone problems often occur at a vulnerable area of the bone, which is individual to each person. Some people have "weak backs," others "sore ankles," others "stiff necks," and on and on. This weakness begins during the ongoing process of bone regeneration. In the core of the bone new cells are generated daily; the health of these cells relies on full nutrient support. But in some areas, let's say your hip, the bone is not regenerating or strengthening at the same rate as the areas above and below the hip. This puts stress on the nerves in this particular area. Also, if you don't have a very strong bone structure, due to a past break or sprain, the bone tends to bend or move out of normal alignment; this too puts pressure on nerves and muscle structures—all causing pain.

There are several reasons you may have vulnerable bone areas. Lack of proper nutrition is the most common cause of many of today's musculoskeletal problems. Also, the bone you broke years ago may have caused that bone area to become vulnerable to weakness and pain. (In other instances, a vulnerable bone may break and, if healed properly, may become stronger than before!) Almost any injury, disease, or ailment can affect the regeneration of bone cells and result in a vulnerable area that will give you chronic trouble.

MUSCULAR PAIN

There are three common causes of chronic muscle pain: muscles that are out of sync with skeletal structure, muscle stretching, and muscle breakage.

Muscles fall out of alignment with the skeletal structure in many ways. The shoes you wear, the way you walk, the way you sit, your posture, your exercise habits, and on and on, all affect the position your muscles fall into over the years. Once they move away from their proper place, they may move too close to adjacent nerves, causing chronic pain.

Muscle stretching involves the repetitive or traumatic abuse of a muscle. Muscles often are injured in this way due to lack of exercise and conditioning. The weekend athlete, the overzealous gardener, the seasonal handyman all may suffer the pain of muscle stretching. If improperly treated at the time of its initial occurrence or if an activity repeatedly stretches the same muscle, you may end up with a chronic instability in the area and thus pain.

Torn muscles are relatively uncommon, but they are the source of most chronic muscle pain. Although any muscle can be torn, the calf, hamstring, and shoulder muscles are more prone than others. Surgical repair is required for severe tears; unfortunately, once the muscle has been sewn back together, it cannot regain the positive electrical and circulatory condition that existed prior to the injury. Blockages, weaknesses, and vulnerabilities develop in this area that attract problems, difficulties, and neurological discomforts. The pain of this disruption is chronic and very difficult to treat.

THE MUSCULOSKELETAL PAIN/STRESS CYCLE

Regardless of the location or cause of your musculoskeletal pain, emotional stress can dramatically affect its frequency, intensity, and duration. Emotional stress causes muscular tension that aggravates the pain. As the muscles tense they push against the injured area, putting further pressure on the surrounding nerves. The more your pain is aggravated in this way, the more emotional stress you feel; the more stress—the more pain, and so on around and around in circles. This musculoskeletal pain/stress cycle affects an estimated 40 million Americans and prolongs the pain of musculoskeletal conditions far beyond the expected healing time—causing the original pain syndrome to become a chronic one.

As you'll read later in this chapter, this cycle can be interrupted with psychotherapy and relaxation techniques. But first let's take a look at the conventional approach to musculoskeletal pain.

CONVENTIONAL MEDICINE FOR MUSCULOSKELETAL PAIN

Musculoskeletal pain generally is treated with surgery and/or drug therapy.

Surgery

If you dislocate or break a bone or severely tear a muscle, emergency surgery may be necessary to repair the damage. The pain in these circumstances is acute and should end as the bone or muscle heals. However, for a variety of reasons, sometimes the pain persists long after the damage is healed. Only very rarely can additional surgery remedy this chronic pain.

Drug Therapy

Traditional treatment for musculoskeletal pain often involves the use of over-the-counter drugs (such as aspirin or ibuprofen), prescription drugs, and/or nerve blocks.

The popular over-the-counter medication aspirin (also known as a salicylate) is a relatively safe drug and is most effective in the treatment of various musculoskeletal pain. However, if taken in high doses for long periods of time, it can be quite harmful.

Aspirin abuse can cause gastric irritation, which may lead to ulceration and hemorrhage. It also can affect the liver, cause painless bleeding through the stools (which can result in iron-deficiency anemia), and produce rather frightening symptoms affecting the nervous system such as dizziness, ringing in the ears, drowsiness, visual disturbances, and deafness.

Recognizing the drawbacks of aspirin for pain relief, you might turn to "aspirin-free" pain relievers such as acetaminophen or ibuprofen. Acetaminophen is the active ingredient found in the popular product Tylenol. Unfortunately, acetaminophen does not have the anti-inflammatory action of aspirin that so successfully treats many musculoskeletal disorders. In addition, prolonged use of this drug can be quite harmful to the liver.

Ibuprofen is the active ingredient in the pain relievers Advil, Nuprin, Excedrin IB, and Motrin. Because all of these over-the-counter drugs contain the same active ingredient, you can expect from each of them the same negative side effects. These drugs are irritating to the stomach and intestines and also may produce blurred or diminished vision. Although quite effective for short-term relief, the harmful gastrointestinal effects make ibuprofen a poor choice for chronic pain relief.

All analgesics—aspirin, nonaspirin, prescription, and nonprescription—can cause "rebound" pain. Rebound pain is that pain actually caused by the frequent use of analgesics. When analgesics are taken too often, the body may adapt to having pain relievers in the system at all times. When the pain relief begins to wear off, the awareness of pain becomes greater. When this happens, you either will strengthen the rebound effect by taking more analgesics or will look to stronger, narcotic-based drugs for relief.

Narcotics are useful drugs when used to treat acute pain. However, all narcotics have the potential for causing tolerance, addiction, and withdrawal, and so they are not only inappropriate for long-term use but are dangerous when given over a period of time. Morphine, codeine, and synthetic opiates such as Demerol and methadone are commonly given to relieve musculoskeletal pain, but their addictive quality and serious negative side effects make them problematic to the chronic pain patient.

Barbiturates and tranquilizers have no direct pain-relief action. However, frequently they are prescribed as sleeping aids for patients whose pain keeps them awake at night. These too rapidly produce tolerance and are highly addictive. Many times they are combined with pain-relief medication such as aspirin to serve dual duty—pain reduction and sedation. This combination, however, is dangerous because a person in pain may take more and more pills to gain physical relief, not realizing that the barbiturate/tranquilizer abuse will wreck havoc with the sleep cycle, making it more difficult to sleep, and also cause impairment of judgment and coordination. Additionally, a side effect of habitual barbiturate/tranquilizer use is depression, which can actually increase and prolong pain.

Nerve blocks are another way of delivering drug therapy for musculoskeletal pain. Injections into what are called trigger points offer relief for many who suffer the chronic pain of specific conditions, such as lumbar muscle strain or myofascial syndrome. An injection of a local anesthetic into a specific body point blocks pain messengers from the injured area from reaching the brain.

Although effective, this pharmacological approach to pain relief also has its problems. The relief lasts only as long as or slightly longer than the effects of the anesthesia. If you're an outpatient, this can mean returning to your physician for an injection every day. Also, trigger-point injections treat only the symptom of pain and not the cause, and so the pain always will return. Moreover, because a trigger-point injection can aggravate the condition, often the pain returns with more intensity than before. And finally, the body can develop a tolerance for the anesthesia, requiring more frequent injections with reduced effect.

Because the two mainstays of conventional medicine—surgery and drug therapy—are so often dangerous or ineffective for treating chronic musculoskeletal pain, various kinds of natural medicine are becoming popular alternative additional methods for assisting the millions who suffer "untreatable" musculoskeletal pain.

NATURAL MEDICINE FOR
MUSCULOSKELETAL PAIN

Acupuncture

Acupuncture is an excellent therapy for both bone breaks and muscle injuries. In most cases it can both treat the symptomatic pain and restore the energized flow of *chi* through the body to remove the root cause of the pain.

Treating sports injuries with acupuncture often yields almost miraculous results. Football great Lawrence Taylor tried physical therapy, cortisone shots, and ultrasound treatments before he finally tried acupuncture for a strained left hamstring that had bothered him for months. Athletes who put repetitive stress on certain muscle groups (such as tennis players, runners, and swimmers) are turning to acupuncture more and more frequently to relax muscles before competitions and to relieve severely cramped muscles afterward. Also, when applied immediately, acupuncture is especially effective in treating sprained muscles.

Acupressure

Acupressure can block the transmission of pain impulses by closing the gates of the body's pain-signaling system and by encouraging the release of the body's natural painkillers, endorphins.

Although there are so many sites of musculoskeletal injury it's hard to choose specific local points, self-administered acupressure can be tried by applying firm pressure each day to the following potent points. Don't rub or massage these points, just hold them firmly (without causing pain) for about two or three minutes.

For Upper-Body Musculoskeletal Pain

Li 4: in the webbing between the thumb and index finger at the highest spot of the muscle where the thumb and index finger are brought close together

GB 20: below the base of the skull, in the hollows on either side, two to three inches apart

GB 21: on the highest part of the shoulder

For Lower-Body Muscular Pain

St 36: four finger widths below the kneecap, one finger width outside of the shinbone

K 3: midway between the inside ankle bone and the Achilles' tendon in the back of the ankle

B 60: midway between the outer ankle bone and the Achilles' tendon

Botanical Medicine

For Muscle Pain

The topical application of eucalyptus oil massaged into the sore muscle area will greatly relieve muscular pain. This treatment commonly is applied to the muscle injuries suffered by athletes throughout the world. Eucalyptus oil is available in any health food store, and you also may find it in your local pharmacy.

For Musculoskeletal Pain

A number of herbs have analgesic properties and can be used in place of aspirin. These include *Salix alba* (white willow bark), passionflower, hops, and valerian.

If your pain stems from inflammation in the musculo-skeletal system, you also might talk to your doctor about trying feverfew, which has anti-inflammatory properties.

Chiropractic

For Skeletal Pain

A chiropractor should certainly be on your pain-management team for the control of skeletal pain. When the pain is caused by the bones pushing on adjacent nerves, a chiropractor often can manipulate the bones back into their proper position, away from the nerves, and thus relieve your pain.

For Muscular Pain

Your body is delicately constructed on an axial of gravitational balance. This balance allows the muscles and bones to work in harmony with all other parts of the body and to keep an upright and aligned posture. When this delicate balance is disrupted by injury or disorder, the healthy functioning of the entire body is thrown off, and certain muscle groups may respond to the imbalance with pain. A chiropractor can help you put your musculoskeletal structure back into its proper alignment. This realignment may be enough to take the pressure off a nearby nerve center and resolve your pain problem. In other instances, however, the pain may recur if the muscles habitually return to their improper position. In this case, in addition to your chiro-

practic treatments, you may need to find a physical therapist who is sensitive to the importance of muscular alignment or one practiced in the Rolfing technique of muscular
realignment.

Exercise

Exercise is absolutely wonderful in its ability to remedy
musculoskeletal pain. It works on this pain in many ways:

- Exercise strengthens supportive muscles that hold
  weakened bones and ligaments in place.
- Aerobic exercise increases the level of the body's
  natural painkillers, endorphins.
- The increased oxygen levels resulting from exercise
  improve circulation and the delivery of necessary
  nutrients throughout the body.
- Exercise can enhance the results of a weight-loss
  program geared to taking excess weight off a strained
  musculoskeletal system.
- Exercise offers the psychological benefits of distraction
  and improved self-image.

Different kinds of musculoskeletal conditions require
different kinds of exercise programs. You may need to practice flexibility exercises; others may benefit most from low-
resistance, high-repetition workouts; still others may need
high-resistance, low-repetition exercises. Or you may need
an aerobics program, but you'll need to determine if it
should be a high-impact or low-impact one. Your physician
should be able to suggest appropriate exercises or at least
resources to find them, and of course, a physical therapist
can put you on a therapeutic program.

Homeopathy

Homeopathic medicine is a system you can explore if your muscles seem to injure too easily or too frequently. Whether your problem involves a specific muscle group or simply excessive vulnerability ·to injury, homeopathic care can strengthen the system. The following internal medicines are often prescribed for use three to four times a day, but to be stopped as soon as the pain or stiffness recedes. (However, no treatment should be undertaken without first consulting with your medical professional.)

• *Bryonia 6c* should be considered if motion of the affected joint increases the pain and continuous motion makes the pain more intense.

• *Ruta 6c* is extremely helpful in the treatment of ligaments or tendons that have been torn or wrenched. Ruta should be considered if Rhus tox has not helped or if the injured area does not hurt during initial motion or is relieved by continued motion. Ruta has been known to be effective in the treatment of tennis elbow.

• *Arnica 6c* is by far the most common homeopathic medicine taken for muscular pain. It relieves the pain, reduces swelling, and speeds healing. If the injury is slight, you might simply rub arnica oil onto the affected area. For more severe pain, both the oil and the medicine are used.

• *Rhus tox. 6c* is used to treat muscle injuries due to overexertion.

• *Bellis perennis 6c* might be taken to relieve deep muscle injuries or injuries to the joints, especially if arnica doesn't remedy the problem.

• *Ledum 6c* is a valuable homeopathic remedy for ankle

sprains, particularly when the injured area can be soothed with cold applications.

Hydrotherapy

The use of cold and hot applications for the treatment of musculoskeletal pain is standard practice. Your physician can advise you what kind of hydrotherapy is best suited to your particular pain, but some general statements about the use of hot and cold might help you as you experiment to find the therapy best for you.

Cold-Water Therapy

Ice massage generally is applied immediately after the musculoskeletal injury occurs. Cold reduces circulation, thus reducing the pain and swelling. Cold-water whirlpools also can be used for the same effect.

Warm-Water Therapy

Warm (not hot) compresses, baths, and whirlpools are most appropriate for chronic pain conditions. Warm water increases circulation, relaxes muscles, and relieves muscle spasms.

Hypnosis

Hypnosis has been used successfully in the treatment of musculoskeletal pain. Susceptible patients can be instructed, while under a trance, to feel no pain. Through hypnosis, deep states of relaxation can be attained, allowing tense muscles to relax and blood circulation to flow smoothly, thus easing the pain of tension-based problems. This state of pain relief lasts for a time even after the hypnotic session.

A second use of hypnosis in the treatment of musculoskeletal pain lies in its ability to help you break the muscular habits that can cause or aggravate the pain. While under hypnosis, for example, a patient may be "programmed" to stop limping, slouching, or tensing. In this way the underlying cause of the problem is tackled at the same time the patient may be using other natural therapies to reduce the sensation of pain.

Massage

Massage is a soothing adjunct to other natural remedies in the treatment of chronic musculoskeletal pain. Massage can ease the intensity of chronic pain in three ways: (1) It increases circulation to the affected area, thus improving the oxygen environment; (2) it relaxes the involved muscles and thus interrupts the pain/tension/pain cycle; and (3) increased circulation and relaxed muscles increase the range of motion capable in the affected area.

Nutrition

Bone and muscle pain can be treated with nutritional therapy that strengthens the vulnerable areas. To begin, you need to remove pollutants from your body that increase the acidity level and leave behind waste materials. The most harmful pollutants are caffeine, alcohol, and nicotine. If you feel you are addicted to coffee, alcohol, or cigarettes, talk to your doctor about how you can best break the habit to begin nutritional therapy.

Next you'll need to alkalinize your body. Like pollutants,

meats, cheese, white breads, and processed foods also have a high acidity level that leaves waste materials in the body. This waste interferes with the ability of the muscles and bones to absorb the vitamins and minerals they need to remain pain-free. It also blocks the free flow of oxygen that is so necessary to mineral absorption. You can change from this acid state to an alkaline state by replacing these foods with those having a high pH level. Foods such as vegetables, fruits, grains, and beans will do the job. Raw, uncooked alkaline foods further raise the body's pH level because they have oxygen and enzymes that are able to enter the body's cells directly.

Skeletal Pain

Cells develop in the middle of the bone marrow; as the cells age, they move out to become the bone structure itself with the oldest cells forming the outermost part. As new cells develop, their health is based on the amount of nutrition the body provides. If your body is lacking oxygen enzymes, vitamins, and minerals and is overloaded with high-acid and fatty foods, the new cells are weakened and will perpetuate your skeletal pain.

In addition to the alkalinizing diet just suggested, you can treat severe, incessant skeletal pain with apple cider vinegar. This alkalinizes the system rapidly to bring you the quick relief you need from continuous pain. Mix ½ cup of vinegar with ½ cup of juice to make a palatable drink. Take one or more drinks every other day for two weeks and then continue on the alkalinizing diet just outlined.

Psychotherapy

Musculoskeletal pain is quite often difficult to diagnosis precisely and treat effectively. One reason for the difficulty is the number of psychological factors that may be involved. Patients complaining of low-back pain, for example, often are influenced by depression, job dissatisfaction, drug or alcohol abuse, and the prospect of workers' compensation, to name a few.

Because of this close relationship between musculoskeletal pain and psychological factors, psychotherapy is strongly recommended as an integral part of a pain-management program. Exploratory psychotherapy, psychoanalysis, and Gestalt therapy can help patients uncover the root cause of stress, anxiety, or depression that may be finding its release in pain.

Couples therapy and family therapy also are often useful in the treatment of musculoskeletal pain. These kinds of therapies help family members understand the psychological factors involved in musculoskeletal pain and teach them how they may be enabling the pain to continue by unintentionally reinforcing pain behaviors.

Behavioral and cognitive therapies are used quite frequently to treat patients with musculoskeletal pain. In fact, many behavioral psychologists use operant conditioning techniques for those patients who seem resistant to other forms of treatment. This approach to behavior modification rewards desirable behaviors and ignores undesirable ones. One behavioral approach uses exercise, rather than drugs or rest, as a reward for back-pain patients. Patients work toward a specific, attainable exercise goal, such as a given number of repetitions or amount of time on an exercise bicycle; they stop when the goal is attained. This method makes rest (the reward for exercising) dependent on the exercise itself, and not on the experience of pain or fatigue.

Relaxation Techniques

Musculoskeletal pain can be aggravated or even initiated by stress. When you're upset, angry, anxious, or depressed, your muscles tense, your breathing becomes shallow and faster, and the blood flow throughout your body is restricted. All of these physical reactions affect your muscle tension, and this can certainly influence your pain experience. Learning to calm the stress response can help you manage your condition. The following relaxation exercises are suggested as natural remedies for musculoskeletal pain; be sure also to read the full discussion of relaxation and its effect on pain on pages 91–107.

Guided Imagery and Meditation

This relaxation therapy is a useful technique because you can perform it anytime and anywhere.

One type of meditation proven especially helpful uses guided imagery to create movies of the mind. These are short ad-libbed meditations that can reduce pain temporarily. The technique helps you visualize your muscles and bones as healthy and nonpainful in an attempt to "trick" your brain into producing sensations of calm and comfort.

As you feel your pain begin, for example, you might say to yourself:

> *My body is healthy and strong. I feel no pain. My muscles are relaxed and smooth. I can feel rich red blood flow through this area, bringing oxygen and nutrients that keep the pain away. I can see myself walking without pain. I see myself enjoying my life without pain.*

Autogenic Training

Autogenic training can be used to relieve musculoskeletal pain. It enables you to focus your mental energies on particular parts of your body that need to feel calm and warm and healthy.

Deep Breathing

Deep-breathing exercises can stop the body's stress response effectively. This gives you the ability to control the muscle tension that can trigger your pain.

Progressive Muscle Relaxation

Progressive muscle relaxation is an excellent technique for relieving musculoskeletal pain. Once you learn the skill of voluntarily controlling muscular tension, you are able to relax the muscles that aggravate your pain.

Distraction

Although distraction techniques such as music, laughter, and socializing don't stop pain, they do have a place in your pain-management program. When the mind is distracted by other stimuli, it is not able to process persistent pain signals as easily as when you're unoccupied. If you can resist the temptation to take to your bed when your pain begins, you'll find yourself experiencing less discomfort.

Biofeedback

Biofeedback can be used to control musculoskeletal pain. If you find that your pain episodes are worsened by stress, tension, or anxiety, it certainly would be worthwhile to investigate the benefits of this technique. Learning to control your blood pressure and body temperature voluntarily gives you additional control over your pain.

TENS

Transcutaneous electrical nerve stimulation can be used effectively to block the pain signals of musculoskeletal pain.

In addition, TENS is a most remarkably effective treatment for broken bones. Placed at the site of the breakage, the electrical current brings together calcium, magnesium, and other elements to remineralize and thus strengthen that particular area. This therapeutic technique is most effective when applied at the time of the break and is found to be especially beneficial in the treatment of older people whose broken bones don't heal readily by themselves. If, however, you broke a bone even twenty years ago and are still bothered by occasional pain at that bone site, you can use a TENS unit to strengthen that area and relieve the pain permanently.

CHAPTER ELEVEN

Psychogenic Pain

Have you been told that your pain is all in your head? If so, you may be experiencing psychogenic pain—which is not the same thing as saying "You're crazy." The term "psychogenic" means that both the mind and the body are involved in the pain. Given what we know about the interwoven relationship among the mind and body and health, perhaps psychogenic is a term that should be used when speaking of all or any pain. But it is not. Historically, conventional medicine has drawn a line between what is called somatogenic pain, which is pain having a physical, organic cause, and psychogenic pain, which is defined as pain originating in the mind. This distinction has fueled debate between conventional and natural medicine advocates for centuries. Although many medical specialists today recognize the link between physical and psychological pain, psychogenic pain is still problematic for people looking for honest diagnosis and effective treatment.

It's problematic because, realistically, there is no cut-off line between psychological and physical pain. Pure organic pain doesn't exist, because all bodily pain involves an emotional or cognitive response. On the other hand, pure psychogenic pain is also a rarity; the assumption that the true cause of all pain syndromes is known and anything outside those identified conditions is not true pain is unwarranted because the physical basis for many pain syndromes is unclear. Recent advances in diagnostic radiology have pinpointed physical bases for syndromes that, prior to the development of such sophisticated technology, were thought to be of psychological origin.

Still, despite this logical and rational basis for categorizing psychogenic pain as "true" pain, the term carries many negative connotations. Associated with the diagnosis of psychogenic pain are stereotypes including "hypocondria" or "hysteria," and even personality descriptors such as "demanding" or "manipulative." For you, the task of proving your pain can become more complicated and emotionally draining than the pain itself. Most likely you already have invested inordinate amounts of time and money looking for a reason for your pain, all the while suffering from pain that you're told is "all in your head."

In the search for the pain's source, the word "psychogenic" is often confused with other terms. The word "psychosomatic," for example, frequently is used interchangeably with "psychogenic" by both the general public and members of the medical community. The difference between the two is subtle but notable. "Psychosomatic" refers to a disease state that is *influenced* by the mind—ulcers, colitis, and some allergies, for example. "Psychogenic" refers to a disease state that is *caused* by the mind—having no roots in any physical disease or disorder. Also, the word "hypochondriac" is frequently used to label those suffering psychogenic pain. Hypochondria is quite different but more difficult to define. Although the medical literature lacks an acceptable definition of hypochondria, there is general agreement that the person with hypochondriacal neurosis is characterized as having a preoccupation with his or her body and a constant fear of disease and body malfunction. It has been found that the patient with pain as a hypochondriacal symptom focuses a great deal on the pain and its origin but exhibits no marked anxiety or depression such as frequently accompanies psychogenic pain.

THE ROOTS OF
PSYCHOGENIC PAIN

Pain of psychogenic origin can grow from innumerable psychological conflicts, including personal, interpersonal, marital, familial, occupational, and spiritual ones. But as a whole, they can be categorized into four relatively well-defined subgroups: (1) pain as a symptom of depression, (2) pain as a symptom of anxiety, (3) pain as a symptom of hysterical neurosis, and (4) pain as a symptom of unresolved grief.

Pain as a Symptom of Depression

Because depression often is accompanied by heightened self-concern and awareness of the body, pain complaints are common in clinical depression. Unfortunately, too often the focus of treatment falls on the pain, rather than on the true cause—the depression.

If you suspect that your pain is psychogenic, you can identify depression as its root by asking yourself these questions:

- Have you been feeling "down" lately?
- Do you become fatigued easily?
- Have you been having trouble concentrating?
- Have you lost interest and satisfaction in work?
- Are you unable to function efficiently?
- Have you withdrawn from family and friends?

- Do you have unprovoked crying spells?
- Have you been experiencing sleep disturbances, constipation, loss of weight or appetite, or decreased interest in sex?
- Have you thought about suicide?

A "yes" answer to any one of these questions indicates the possibility of depression and the need to consider it as the source of your pain.

Pain as a symptom of depression also should be considered based on your past history. This pain syndrome may be found in those who have experienced past depressions (particularly those that required hospitalization), have a history of alcoholism or accident-proneness, and have had previous episodes of hyperactivity or manic behavior. If any of these are a part of your past, you might consider depression as the cause of your pain.

Which Came First—the Depression or the Pain?

When a pain complaint is coupled with symptoms of depression, it's not always easy to tell if the pain is psychogenic or somatogenic. Like patients experiencing psychogenic pain, patients suffering pain such as arthritis or neuralgia with an identified physical source may show many of the symptoms of depression. That's why the true diagnostic task is to determine whether the patient is suffering psychogenic pain caused by the depression or is experiencing depression secondary to chronic pain. Making the distinction is critical to successful management and is done by establishing when the depression first occurred. If the depression seems to have existed before the pain, you can assume it's psychogenic pain. Because it is not always easy to pinpoint the onset of depression, determining which came first—the pain or the depression—can be difficult. Careful history-taking and attention to all events in your life at or near the time the complaint originated is most helpful in making an accurate diagnosis.

Pain as a Symptom of Anxiety

Like depression, anxiety also can cause heightened body awareness. Acute anxiety frequently is accompanied by a vague sense of fearfulness that brings on exaggerated concern over medical symptoms.

When anxiety increases, some people subconsciously may begin to hyperventilate. Hyperventilation sets off a series of reactions—deficiency of carbon dioxide and a change in the acid/base balance in the blood, resulting in changes in the ratio of bound to unbound calcium, and, finally, neuromuscular disturbances. Among the most commonly seen neuromuscular symptoms are a feeling of impending doom; tingling around the mouth, hands, and feet; an inability to catch one's breath; and often acute chest pain.

Psychogenic chest pain caused by anxiety is easily confused with angina pain. As with the pain/depression relationship, only careful consideration of your history and life events surrounding the onset of pain can distinguish the two. Misdiagnosis leads to mistreatment; therefore, it's important for you to determine which appeared first—the pain or the anxiety. Angina pain comes on suddenly and then is followed by feelings of anxiety; psychogenic chest pain follows a period of anxiety.

Pain as a Symptom of Hysterical Neurosis

Sometimes pain symptoms represent attempts to resolve personal conflict that a person cannot deal with in a healthy way. Such symptoms are rooted in hysterical neuroses and are sometimes called conversion symptoms. The symptoms of hysterical neuroses are goal-oriented. A particular pain, for example, might make it impossible for you to carry out a certain task or role that you don't want to be responsible for. Other typical characteristics of this kind of psychogenic problem might include: (1) pain description that relates to an underlying personal conflict; (2) indifference to the pain despite its continued presence; (3) sudden onset of pain in an emotionally charged situation; (4) pain description that defies the facts of human physiology; and (5) evidence of benefits gained because of the pain (that is, desired release from responsibilities or gratification in dependency).

Any personal or interpersonal conflict can cause conversion symptoms (of which pain is becoming the most common), provided the patient can neither consciously face the dilemma nor accept the responsibilities that healthy resolution of the conflict would impose. Typical conflictual settings include marital discord and other family and sex-related problems, job difficulties, and nonrecovery from traumatic injury, particularly where there are disability or compensation issues.

Pain as a Symptom of Unresolved Grief

It is normal and necessary to experience grief and mourning following the death of a close relative or friend. In its normal course, the grieving process brings bereaved people through different stages until finally the grief is resolved and they have the desire and ability to get on with their lives. If you are unable to grieve at all or to work through the entire grieving process, you are at increased risk for suffering pain as a symptom of grief.

Diagnosis of this kind of pain requires an honest appraisal of the grieving process. Unresolved grief should be strongly suspected as the cause of your pain if you have sought medical help for symptoms similar to those of the deceased, if the pain appeared shortly after the death of a loved one, if you still feel that the loss is too painful to talk about, or if you feel a need but an inability to cry.

These are four possible sources of psychogenic pain that you might consider if you have a pain complaint that doctors say has no basis in a physical problem. Unfortunately, when a pain has no basis in a physical problem, there is an implication that there also is no real pain. Rest assured that psychogenic pain is very real, and any accusations of lying or faking are completely invalid.

Indeed, it is difficult to find any difference between a patient of somatogenic pain and a patient of psychogenic pain. Of great interest is the finding that there are no significant differences in psychological test scores between the two groups. Anxious, complaining, and depressive moods are characteristic of both kinds of chronic pain patients. Also, no personality type automatically leads to psychogenic pain complaints.

Psychogenic pain actually serves a valuable function. It is the voice that seeks help for a problem that you yourself have been unable to recognize or talk about. Unfortunately, the cry is too often left unanswered.

CONVENTIONAL MEDICINE
AND THE TREATMENT OF
PSYCHOGENIC PAIN

The belief that all pain must have an organic cause puts psychogenic pain patients at odds with the conventional medical community. When a routine physical examination rules out medical cause for the pain complaint, patients then are frequently subjected to unnecessary and inappropriate medical procedures that become a costly and time-consuming exploratory expedition. Investigative tests, surgeries, and drug dependence become the norm in the treatment of psychogenic pain.

Even when a physician recognizes there may be psychological factors at play, the approach too often falls short of helpful. The case is often dismissed with the pronouncement, "Your pain is probably caused by a psychological problem." The patient is sent home feeling perplexed, embarrassed, angry, and disappointed—and still in pain.

Sometimes physicians who do recognize psychogenic pain syndromes attempt to treat the problem with drug therapy. Various tricyclic antidepressants often are prescribed and may be helpful in lessening the perception of both mental and physical pain. But as is the case with all drug therapies, this can mask the problem and put the patient at risk for serious anticholinergic side effects that can aggravate such clinical conditions as acute angle glaucoma and prostatism, and may induce cardiac arrhythmias. Long-term use can lead to addiction.

Many physicians recognize the relationship between stress and pain. When diagnostic tests fail to find a reason for the pain, they may advise their patients to "relax." Although sometimes this is appropriate advice, it's not enough to help you treat your psychogenic pain. You need specific instructions and guidelines. You need training in relaxation techniques, and you need more detailed information about the interrelationship between the mind and the body. You need the kind of treatments offered through natural medicine therapies.

NATURAL MEDICINE AND THE TREATMENT OF PSYCHOGENIC PAIN

There is no mind/body split in the application of natural medicine. When a functional disorder cannot be found and the practitioners of conventional medicine give up, the natural approach that works within the energetic framework of the body is most effective. Natural medicine can serve to ease psychogenic pain in a number of ways. Some remedies rebalance and unclog the flow of energy throughout the body. Others offer symptomatic relief. Still others deal directly with the psychological root of the pain. A complete description of the following natural therapies is presented in Chapter 3 of this book. Be sure to read this detailed information before using any of the recommended remedies.

Acupuncture

These Oriental therapies are most appropriate in the treatment of psychogenic pain. By reestablishing a balanced flow of *chi*, these remedies can both lessen the pain, and ease the causative mental disruptions.

In Chinese medicine, there is no mind/body split. Each of the meridians is associated with a particular organ or bowel *(zang/fu)*, element, emotion, season, color, and so on. An imbalance of *chi* in a particular meridian or *zang/fu* gives rise to physical, mental, and emotional correlates. Emotions may become causes of disease when they are held over long periods of time, or if they result from something particularly stressful, shocking, or traumatic. Emotions also may result from an imbalance in *chi* flow. They may be either the cause or the symptoms of a disorder. For example, prolonged anger may damage the energetic sphere of the liver, with which it is associated, or imbalance in the energetic sphere of the liver may result in constant anger or, conversely, an inability to feel anger. One of the classics of Chinese medicine, "Simple Questions" describes the effects that various emotions have on *chi* flow:

Anger makes Chi rise and causes vomiting of Blood and diarrhea.

Joy makes the Mind peaceful and relaxed, it benefits the Nutritive and Defensive Chi and it makes Chi relax and slow down.

Sadness makes the Heart cramped and agitated, this pushes towards the Lungs' lobes, the Upper Burner becomes obstructed, Nutritive and Defensive Chi cannot circulate freely. Heat accumulates and dissolves Chi.

Fear depletes the Essence, it blocks the Upper Burner, which makes Chi descend to the Lower Burner.

Shock affects the Heart, depriving it of residence, the Mind has no shelter and cannot rest, so that Chi becomes chaotic.

We have all experienced this in our lives. The sinking feeling we feel when afraid; the tightening of our neck and shoulders when angry, sometimes accompanied by the desire to strike out; and the slowing down of time when we are happy. What Chinese medicine is saying is that our emotions affect the flow of *chi*, and if we are habitually stressed in a certain way, our *chi* becomes habituated to that manner of flowing. As a result, tension develops in the musculature associated with these areas of the body, and this tension in turn has an effect on the organs and viscera in the area of the body involved. For example, someone who is constantly angry may suffer ailments associated with having too much *chi* in the upper portion of the body: for example, hypertension or migraines.

Acupuncture can be a very effective therapy for the treatment of stress-related disorders because it is able to redirect the flow of *chi* into a more normal and balanced flow. Acupuncture helps to retrain the *chi* to flow in its balanced, unstressed pattern. Acupuncture also provides support to the underlying energetic spheres affected, helping to resolve the cause or the effects of stress. From a Western perspective, acupuncture releases tension in the muscles, and this in turn allows increased flow of blood, lymph, and nerve impulses to the affected areas. This helps decrease the stress experienced. Of course, acupuncture also is very effective in relieving the physical symptoms that may be associated with stress disorders, such as insomnia, headaches, neck and shoulder tension, nausea, diarrhea, heart palpitations, and so on.

The specific course of treatment depends on the pattern of your symptoms and their severity. Acupuncture treatment for anxiety, for example, may last approximately ten to twelve weeks, with one session per week.

Botanical Medicine

Herbalism can be used to treat the depression that can be the underlying cause of some psychogenic pain. *Hypericum perforatum* has been prescribed as an antidepressant. This herb encourages the release of serotonin in the brain, which promotes natural feelings of well-being.

Chiropractic

Because some psychological problems have physical components, chiropractic can be an effective adjunct therapy in the treatment of psychogenic pain. Through chiropractic manipulation, a practitioner can offer symptomatic relief of pain, tension, and stress. This therapy may not remedy psychogenic pain by itself, but it can be used along with other forms of natural medicine to ease the pain of this complex condition.

Exercise

There are no exercises developed specifically to relieve psychogenic pain. Still, exercise should be a component of your pain-management program because of its overall healing effects.

Aerobic exercise, such as walking or bicycling, which increases the rate of your heartbeat, is especially beneficial because it:

• promotes mineral absorbtion in the body, which can help correct nutritional imbalances that cause or aggravate your pain

• increases the oxygen content of the blood; this improves circulation and the delivery of nutrients to all parts of the body

• keeps muscles strong and flexible, which reduces the pain caused by muscle tension and stiffness

• triggers the release of the body's natural painkillers, endorphins

As a natural therapy, exercise is a wonderful relaxation strategy and diversionary tactic. Use it regularly along with the other natural remedies you choose for your pain-management program.

Homeopathy

Homeopathy can treat psychogenic pain successfully when the psychological root cause is established. However, because successful use of homeopathy becomes a matter of your specific constitutional state, treatment is best left to a trained homeopathic professional.

Hydrotherapy

Depending on the location of the pain, hydrotherapy can be used to treat the symptoms of psychogenic pain.

Inflamed, swollen areas are best treated with cold therapies such as baths or ice massage. These restrict the flow of blood to the area and reduce the pain.

Chronic pain without inflammation is best treated with hot or warm therapies such as whirlpools, baths, and heating pads. Heat brings more blood into the painful area; this improves circulation, delivers more oxygen and nutrients, and carries away toxic waste.

Hydrotherapy can offer symptomatic relief for many psychogenic pain syndromes, but be sure to check with your physician before applying any heat or cold to your pain area. Used incorrectly, heat or cold also can aggravate the problem.

Hypnosis

Hypnosis is used in the treatment of psychogenic pain in several ways. It can ease pain exacerbated by stress, tension, or anxiety by leading you into a deep state of relaxation. It also can help you disassociate from the pain, thereby lessening the perception of pain. And it can be used as a therapeutic tool to help you find the psychological root of the pain. Under hypnosis, many people have been able to uncover deeply hidden mental traumas that have found outlet in pain. Once uncovered, the pain, which has lost its purpose, may subside.

Massage and Reflexology

Massage and reflexology promote relaxation and general body healing. These soothing therapies can be helpful to psychogenic pain patients when used together with other natural medicine modalities.

Nutrition

Pain that is diagnosed as psychogenic can be remedied through nutritional therapy in two ways. First there exists the possibility that a lack of minerals is the actual cause of pain; because this root of chronic pain is not generally identified through conventional diagnostic measures, the pain may be categorized as psychogenic.

Second, when pain truly is a symptom of psychological conflict, the fact is that the mind would be unable to use pain as this kind of diversionary tactic unless there existed a vitamin and mineral imbalance.

In both cases, the pain can be reduced or eliminated by changes in your diet that increase the B vitamins and minerals, especially calcium, magnesium, mineral salts, iron, and copper.

Increase your B vitamins by eating whole-grain products such as breads, muffins, and long-grain rice. B vitamins also are found in most vegetables, including beans.

Increase your calcium and magnesium intake with celery, alfalfa sprouts, kale, nori (a sea vegetable) and dulse tablets and kelp tablets.

Your susceptibility to pain greatly increases through a lack of iron because this reduces the presence of vitamin B_{12} in the body. B_{12} deficiency causes multiple problems, including easy bruising and nerve damage. Unfortunately, the iron supplements often taken to remedy this problem do not work; isolated from other vitamins and minerals, they are not absorbed into the body and cause heavy metal toxicity in many people. A good source of iron can be found in beets and in dulse tablets and kelp tablets.

Increase your copper intake with pumpkin seeds, almonds, and sunflower seeds.

Supplements alone will not improve the imbalance that allows the pain of psychogenic origin to become chronic. Use natural foods to nourish your body and eliminate your pain.

Psychotherapy

If you have psychogenic pain, then you certainly know that guilt and shame accompany this diagnosis. Your doctor has probably told you to "relax"; your family may be impatient and insist "There's nothing wrong with you"; and you yourself may think you're going crazy because you suffer endlessly from something you can't prove even exists. At this time you don't need to be talked out of your pain—you need to be believed. Psychotherapy is an important component of your natural approach to treating your kind of pain.

Cognitive-Behavioral Therapy

This kind of psychological therapy will help you understand that the way you think about your pain influences the way you react to it. If you see yourself as a victim who must give up your physical and social activities, you'll dramatically diminish the quality of your life. Cognitive-behavioral therapy will help you identify your negative thought patterns and behaviors and replace them with positive ones that put you in control and reward your efforts.

Couples and Family Therapy

When you suffer psychogenic pain, your family suffers too. They too are confused and frustrated over the physical and emotional pain you feel, and they may be feeling angry about the time and money you've invested in this ailment that "doesn't exist." Couples and family therapy can help all of you better deal with psychogenic ailments as real medical conditions that need more care and understanding.

Supportive Psychotherapy

The psychogenic pain patient needs supportive therapy because only someone who has experienced this dilemma of pain without cause can understand the physical and mental anguish involved. Supportive therapy gives you a place to talk about your pain, share your feelings, and gain practical advice and insight. Ask your doctor or therapist to help you locate a support group in your area.

Exploratory Psychotherapy

Psychoanalysis and Gestalt therapy can help you understand underlying conflicts of your psychogenic pain. Pain as a symptom of depression, anxiety, conversion, or grief sometimes requires that the source be uncovered and confronted.

In traditional insight-oriented therapies, the client is helped to understand how the problematic factors in his or her life interrelate. As one deepens this kind of understanding, the psychological underpinnings of pain (for example) are seen, and this can result in an alleviation of this symptom. Unfortunately, there is no guarantee that getting more insight into your problems will alleviate the discomfort you feel.

Relaxation Techniques

Stress and anxiety are commonly at the root of psychogenic pain. Relaxation therapy is a useful adjunct in the management of this pain in two ways: It can help you calm the tension that may be causing your pain, and it also can teach you how to interrupt the physical stress reactions that aggravate the pain as it exists now.

In addition to the following brief overview, be sure to read the details in Chapter 3 that explain exactly how relaxation can help alleviate pain.

Psychogenic pain is especially vulnerable to the pain cycle: The more it hurts, the more you worry about it; the more you worry about it, the more it hurts. Distraction tactics such as music, laughter, and socializing can divert your attention away from the pain and therefore change your perception of its intensity.

The relaxation therapies of meditation, deep breathing, and guided visual imagery also are effective in managing psychogenic pain. The calm state generated through these strategies has helped many patients reduce their psychological tensions and thus their pain.

Autogenic training and progressive muscle relaxation are both relaxation techniques that can be used to reduce the pain and the muscular tension that may be causing your pain. These strategies are especially helpful for musculoskeletal pain.

Biofeedback is a relaxation therapy that will give you a sense of control over your emotions and bodily responses. This sense of power can be very effective in helping you gain the psychological upper ground you need to work your way out of your pain. Biofeedback also is a way of connecting some bodily functions so as to mitigate pain.

TENS

Transcutaneous electrical nerve stimulation can be used to interrupt the pain signal of psychogenic pain. However, it cannot address the root cause or help you find the state of relaxation and peace that will silence the nagging pain of mental anguish.

CHAPTER TWELVE

Pain in the Elderly

Has your doctor told you that your pain is to be expected because you're over age sixty? That sometimes happens because biased beliefs about the aging process cause chronic pain in the elderly to be judged on a scale quite different from that used to evaluate pain in the general population. Pain in the elderly, so the myth goes, is a normal part of aging—something to be expected and treated passively with a grin-and-bear attitude. True, you may experience more pain syndromes than most, but much of the pain associated with old age is not inevitable or unmanageable.

The prevalence of chronic benign pain among the elderly is virtually unknown. But a sampling can be drawn from recent research studies such as "A Survey of Chronic Pain in an Elderly Population," printed in the *Canadian Family Physician*. It reported that a recent study of 132 elderly subjects found 83 percent had some form of pain-related problem.

Elderly people frequently suffer from a variety of chronic pain conditions. Physicians report that headaches seem to be the most common pain complaint from their elderly patients. Chronic head pain may indeed be related to aging and caused by vision changes and vascular changes in general. Neuralgia (pain in the distribution of a sensory nerve) and myalgia (pain from skeletal muscle) also com-

monly cause pain problems for the elderly, along with arthritis and lower back pain associated with aging. Other
pain syndromes known to affect the elderly population dis-
proportionately include herpes zoster, temporal arteritis,
and cancer. Some of these conditions have an organic origin and others stem from psychogenic roots, but in either
case, the pain is real and the suffering should not be
chalked up to "being old."

Side Effects of Chronic Pain

The problem of dealing with your pain is not confined to
the pain itself (as many conventional physicians seem to
believe). Similar to its effect on the general population, the
presence of chronic pain at your age is associated with depression, sleep disturbance, overuse of medication, and increased health-care use and medical costs. Particular to
your age group, chronic pain also causes falls, slow rehabilitation, difficulty in movement, impaired mental functioning, and malnutrition.

In addition to the physical ramifications of chronic pain,
you also might suffer emotional reactions that reduce your
ability to participate in the activities of daily life. When
chronic pain is immobilizing, it decreases socialization and
might lead you to become preoccupied with yourself and
your pain. It's not unusual that reactions of anger and loneliness often follow; ultimately you may find that your pain
and your reaction to it have disrupted your family relationships and support systems.

All of these side effects of chronic pain clearly affect the
quality of life in its final stages.

PROBLEMS IN DIAGNOSING
CHRONIC PAIN IN
THE ELDERLY

You can make it difficult for physicians to assess and treat your pain. This difficulty occurs because beliefs about aging often affect how you perceive your pain, what information you tell others, and what activities you're willing to engage in. For example, elderly patients often choose to underreport their pain when they:

- fear their pain is a sign of progressing disease

- are weary of medical testing and doctor bills

- have handed responsibility for their health over to family members and resent the loss of control in decision making

- suffer multiple illnesses and fear accusations of hypochondria

- fear the loss of control and negative side effects caused by the narcotic drugs that are repeatedly prescribed to reduce pain complaints

- want to avoid invasive and unfamiliar procedures such as intubation and spinal taps

Because chronic pain in the elderly is not easily understood, information about this aspect of geriatric medicine has been extrapolated from experience with younger patients and those with cancer pain. This lack of focus on the chronic pain of the elderly leaves the conventional medical community with a narrow and sometimes dangerous approach to managing pain in the elderly population.

CONVENTIONAL MEDICINE IN
THE TREATMENT OF PAIN
IN THE ELDERLY

Analgesic drug therapy is the treatment of choice for pain control in the elderly. You may be prescribed either nonsteroidal anti-inflammatory drugs (NSAIDs) such as aspirin or ibuprofen or opiate analgesic drugs such as morphine or codeine. Antidepressants, anticonvulsants, and sedatives also are often prescribed to relieve the anxiety, stress, and tension associated with chronic pain. Drug therapy does give short-term pain relief, but as detailed in Chapter 1, it can cause very undesirable side effects when used to treat chronic conditions. These drugs pose additional problems when used by senior members of the population.

Adverse effects that have been associated with NSAID use among the elderly population include peptic ulcer disease, renal insufficiency, and bleeding diathesis. These problems give you reason to question the overall safety of NSAIDs for the treatment of your pain.

Opiate analgesics also present a unique set of side effects specific to the elderly. For example, if a drug causes sedation, disorientation, or confusion, your risk for injury from falls is greatly increased. This potential for falls was highlighted in a study of seventy-four institutionalized elderly people. In their study "Falls Among the Institutionalized Elderly," Perlin and associates reported that at the time of falls, 60 patients (81 percent) were taking central nervous system drugs and 58 (78 percent) were taking nonsteroidal anti-inflammatory drugs.

Xerostomia, or dry mouth, is another common side effect of narcotic use in the elderly. Dry mouth can cause taste impairment, difficulty with eating dry foods and with speech and swallowing. Denture wearers may have additional problems such as denture sores, denture retention, and the tongue sticking to the palate.

Many elderly patients fear any drug therapy that can affect their cognitive functioning. You may be concerned about age-related memory loss, confusion, and disorientation and therefore should be leery of any pain treatment that will exacerbate these problems. Also, because of an enhanced sensitivity to drugs, even moderate drug use can cause you nightmares, anxiety, agitation, euphoria, dysphoria, paranoia, hallucinations, and depression.

Other side effects of opiate analgesics include:

* respiratory depression
* constipation
* paradoxical effects
* sexual problems including erectile problems, vaginal dryness, impotence, ejaculatory abnormalities, and decreased libido
* addiction

Dr. Bruce Ferrell, assistant professor of medicine/geriatrics at the UCLA School of Medicine, has reported that three particular opiate drugs deserve special mention because of their potential to cause problems in the elderly.

Propoxyphene hydrochloride (Darvon) is a controversial drug that is probably overprescribed in the elderly. Controlled trials suggest that its efficacy is no better than aspirin or acetaminophen, and it has significant potential for addiction as well as renal injury.

Pentazocine (Talwin) is an opiate drug that should be avoided because it frequently causes delirium and agitation in the elderly.

Long-acting opiates such as methadone should be used

with extreme caution because of the propensity for drug accumulation in the frail elderly.

Some of these side effects can be minimized with careful attention to the properties of the drug and its effect on the aged. For example, knowing that elderly patients are more sensitive to the pain-relieving properties of opiate drugs than are younger patients, physicians can reduce the likelihood of addiction and drug accumulation by reducing the dosage prescribed. Thus, you may achieve pain relief from smaller doses of opiate drugs compared to younger patients.

Physicians also must be aware that the side effects of drug therapy can be compounded by the fact that the elderly patient is very likely to be using medication for other conditions such as diabetes, heart disease, hypertension, or arthritis. Physiological changes that normally accompany the aging process alter absorption, distribution, excretion, and drug metabolism. This phenomenon increases your predisposition to adverse effects from multiple medications.

Drug therapy for the treatment of pain in the elderly offers a narrow approach to your pain: It tries to treat the symptom as if it existed as a separate entity from your emotional, spiritual, and mental health. In the treatment of the elderly, where pain is wrongly considered inevitable and responsive only to passive treatment with drugs, alternative treatment remedies are most especially welcomed.

NATURAL MEDICINE FOR THE TREATMENT OF PAIN IN THE ELDERLY

Drug therapy certainly has its place in the treatment of your chronic pain. But without a doubt, pain management can be improved by taking the primary focus off medication and turning the emphasis toward natural therapies. The holistic approach will give you a different perspective on your pain, encompassing not only the physical aspects of pain, but also mental and social aspects so often overlooked by family, friends, and physicians. In addition, this approach more realistically meets your needs if you also are struggling with depression.

Depression in the elderly is greatly complicated by the psychological, social, and emotional components of chronic pain. If your needs as a total person are ignored, you're more likely to feel worried, frightened, helpless, hopeless, angry, or even suicidal. That's why things such as the fear of death and the loss of function, self-esteem, and independence that accompany chronic pain must be addressed in the pain-management program.

The natural therapies recommended in this book are particularly appropriate for you because they require active involvement. When you take responsibility for your own pain relief, you're more likely to feel your pain is manageable because you're doing something about it for yourself. From exercise to psychotherapy, natural medicine offers noninvasive techniques that can help you manage your pain.

A brief summation of natural remedies that have been found to be useful in the management of pain in the elderly follows. In addition, be sure to review the complete description of these therapies presented in Chapter 3.

Acupuncture and Acupressure

Acupuncture is a two-thousand-year-old Chinese technique of inserting fine needles into the skin at selected body points. The insertion of needles is believed to remove any blocks to the body's energy flow and thus restore harmony. Acupressure is a less invasive procedure that uses finger pressure and massage at acupuncture sites. Both therapies can relieve many types of chronic pain, especially pain associated with headaches, arthritis, neuralgia, lower back, and other musculoskeletal problems.

Much of Chinese medicine and acupuncture was based on maintaining the health of the emperor and increasing longevity. Therefore, much attention has been paid to encouraging the flow of energy and preventing the occurrence of the usual discomforts associated with aging such as pain, stiffness, and decreasing vitality. When such problems do exist, acupuncture helps not only with pain but with digestive problems, stress management, and other difficulties by nurturing the vital essences.

With more education and acceptance, the American public has begun to use acupuncture and acupressure for difficult-to-diagnose energetic problems and also for health maintenance and preventive care.

Botanical Medicine

Botanical medicine uses plants and herbs to treat specific ailments and assist recuperation from illness in order to restore physiological balance.

Botanical remedies have been found to relieve any pain that can be treated conventionally with aspirin or steroids. For pain relief talk to your doctor about trying *Salix alba* (white willow bark), passionflower, hops, and valerian.

For pain that's accompanied by inflammation (as is likely to be the case with arthritis, musculoskeletal problems, and lower back pain), try feverfew. This contains anti-inflammatory properties.

Chiropractic

Chiropractic medicine involves spinal manipulations that can adjust specific vertebrae in order to remove any interference with nerves. It also may involve a general manipulation of bones in order to realign joints and increase range of motion.

Chiropractic medicine can be applied to relieve many pain syndromes including: lower back and disk problems, neuralgias arising in the spinal column and the pelvis, postural defects causing muscle pain, sprains and strains of the rib cage, traumatic bursitis or tendonitis, and functional disorders of the internal organs and systems that are consequences of mechanical irritation of nerve pathways.

Maintaining the body in equilibrium through spinal manipulation also can help increase the strength of the immune system. By relaxing tense muscles and increasing circulation, chiropractic medicine promotes a stronger and healthier body system.

Exercise

Lack of physical activity is a major problem affecting pain management in the elderly. Pain behaviors such as excessive bed rest and limited physical movement increase the perception of pain and contribute to the pain of physical deterioration. In addition, loss of muscle mass associated with the aging process may by itself be the basis for some pain. Other elders may experience pain related to problems affecting their posture and gait.

Fortunately, exercise is a highly effective therapeutic approach to these problems. Exercise releases endorphins, which can raise your pain threshold. It also contributes to improved physical functioning, strength, flexibility, and range of motion. And it has a positive effect on sleep, appetite, mood, and general health.

The kind of exercise program most appropriate for individual pain conditions will vary. A program focusing on stretching and strengthening specific muscles and joints may be useful in managing musculoskeletal pain and enhancing functional activity. An aerobic exercise program is useful for treating headache, backache, TMJ, and any other kind of pain that is aggravated by stress and tension.

Of course, the degree of physical activity must be tailored to your level of physical fitness. If years of relative inactivity have left your muscles and bones weak and/or unstable, safe and effective conditioning and rehabilitation may be best accomplished with the help of a physical therapist.

Hydrotherapy

Hydrotherapy uses hot, warm, and/or cold water to relieve a variety of pain complaints. Heat treatments dilate blood vessels to improve blood circulation to the affected area. Cold treatments constrict swollen blood vessels to relieve pain and inflammation. Hydrotherapy can be used effectively to treat the pain of arthritis, back pain, musculoskeletal pain, and even psychogenic pain.

Hydrotherapy often is especially helpful in treating the elderly because, for a variety of reasons, circulation becomes restricted with age. Hot and cold therapy can alleviate this problem.

Hypnosis

Hypnosis produces a trancelike state in which you can achieve relief through altered perceptions of pain. Through hypnosis, deep states of relaxation can be attained, allowing tense muscles to relax and blood circulation to flow smoothly, thus easing the pain of tension-based problems. Hypnosis is particularly renowned in its use in treating pain of psychogenic origin. Through hypnosis, patients can identify the psychological source of distress and thereby relieve or even eliminate the physical pain.

Massage

Swedish massage employs continuous, rhythmic motions on the soft tissues, muscles, and ligaments of the body. It stimulates circulation and the function of the nervous system. It is most beneficial in reducing pain caused by stress and muscle tension.

Nutrition

Many pain syndromes in the elderly are caused by a breakdown in the system due to poor nutritional habits developed over the years. Fortunately, it's never "too late" to break these habits and halt the breakdown process.

As you'll read in the other chapters on specific pain problems, most ailments either are caused or are exacerbated by pollutants and foods with high acidity levels. A general nutritional program that can alkalinize your body and reduce, or even eliminate, your pain is as follows:

- Eliminate pollutants such as coffee, black tea, cigarettes, and alcohol.
- Eliminate foods high in fat and sugar content.
- Eliminate acid-based foods such as meats, cheese, white breads, and processed foods.

- Increase your intake of alkalinizing foods such as vegetables, fruits, grains, and beans.
- Begin a supervised exercise program to improve the body's ability to absorb nutrients in an enriched oxygen environment.

Psychotherapy

Cognitive-Behavioral Therapy

Cognitive-behavioral therapy should be an integral component of your pain-management program. Your beliefs about pain and your reactions to those beliefs have an astounding influence on the way you perceive pain. Cognitive therapy can help identify the mental beliefs that keep the pain syndrome in full swing; and it is particularly helpful in debunking the myths surrounding pain and the elderly.

Behavioral therapy focuses on the way you act in response to certain situations. This therapy will help you identify and change pain behaviors such as excessive bed rest, social isolation, abandonment of simple responsibilities, and passive acceptance of pain.

Couples and Family Therapy

Couples and family therapy can be very helpful for you and your family. Family members often unknowingly contribute to the pain experience; they may become tired of hearing about your pain and so avoid conversation completely; others may take over all household responsibilities and insist that you "rest" to avoid aggravating the pain.

Spouses and family members often have trouble dealing with their own emotions of anger, resentment, and fears that are inflamed by living with a chronic pain sufferer. And loved ones too may perpetuate the myth that says "Pain goes with aging and it's something that we all have to accept." Couples and family therapy eases these additional stresses and misunderstandings that compound the chronic pain experience. The results of couples and family support, education, and therapy can dramatically influence the effectiveness of most chronic pain management remedies.

Supportive Therapy

You may have few opportunities to talk about your pain experiences. You may be widowed, or have lost close friends, or feel your infirmity is a burden on your family and so decide to handle it in silence. In these circumstances, supportive group therapy is exceptionally effective in helping you cope with your pain. Sharing both fears and accomplishments with people who empathize and understand is motivational and comforting.

Psychoanalysis

It is not at all uncommon for pain symptoms in the elderly to serve as a release for psychological distress. Retirement, illness of a spouse, death of a spouse or friends, financial difficulties, fear of death, lifelong regrets, and so on often plague members of this population. Psychoanalysis can help uncover the root of pain symptoms, and the therapist can offer coping techniques to help you deal with any underlying problem and thus relieve your pain.

Reflexology

Reflexology is the technique of deeply massaging the soles of the feet (and sometimes the hands) in order to affect various parts of the body therapeutically. Practitioners believe that internal organs share the same nerve supplies as certain corresponding areas of the skin; therefore, pressing the proper points on the feet can stimulate the organ associated with that point.

Reflexology is most beneficial for functional pain disorders that can be reversed, such as headaches and back pain.

Relaxation Techniques

Relaxation techniques are very effective in treating chronic pain in the elderly. Relaxation strategies can influence blood pressure, heart rate, respiration, and metabolism. They can decrease muscle tension and relieve anxiety. They even can promote restful sleep. All of these bodily functions are involved in the pain syndrome and are often of special concern to people over age sixty. Relaxation techniques can even activate the release of the body's own natural painkillers.

A major benefit of relaxation techniques is that the exercises are active, self-administered therapies. Once the techniques have been learned, they can be used throughout the day at your discretion without depending on anyone else; they are minimally time-consuming and low risk, and they provide a sense of control over the pain. (See Chapter 3 for a discussion of specific relaxation techniques.)

TENS

Transcutaneous electrical nerve stimulation is an appropriate and effective treatment modality for most pain. This pain-management technique often is underused for geriatric patients because of various concerns about decreased skin sensation or hypersensitivity. But the results of a study and a review of research literature presented in the article "TENS and Geriatrics" reported in *Clinical Management* found no significant difference between TENS treatment parameters and utilization for individuals under age sixty and individuals sixty years of age or older. In fact, a questionnaire compiled to predict the type of patient most responsive to TENS treatment revealed the ideal type of patient to be a retired and elderly individual. Another clinical study of more than 230 individuals receiving TENS treatment reported that patients over the age of fifty-six years benefited from treatment to a higher degree (21 percent more) than did those age fifty-five or younger.

Ask your doctor about transcutaneous electrical nerve stimulation. It may be the source of pain relief you've been looking for.

Many natural, noninvasive remedies can be used effectively to manage pain in the elderly. Most notable about a natural approach to pain relief for this population is that it really is no different from that suggested for younger chronic pain patients. The treatment of chronic pain and its accompanying depression in the elderly requires the same comprehensive and holistic approach that addresses biological, psychological, social, and familial perspectives.

Chapter Thirteen

Pain Clinics

Here in this last chapter, you'll find that there's a place where many of the natural therapies are brought together into one supervised program. Certainly, you can implement the remedies on your own or with a trained, private therapist, but you also can seek out the help of a pain-management team at a pain clinic.

During the past decade, the pain clinic has become a popular alternative to the conventional treatment of persistent pain. "The idea that pain can sometimes be a disease in itself revolutionized treatment in the 1980s," says Dr. Sridhar Vasudevan, president of the American Academy of Pain Medicine. Now hundreds of accredited clinics specialize in chronic pain and employ a variety of therapies, all emphasizing pain management rather than cures.

INPATIENT AND OUTPATIENT CLINICS

Pain clinics are structured in a variety of ways. They may be private or public, inpatient or outpatient. Most operate primarily out of large, university-affiliated medical centers and are organized as time-limited inpatient programs. Inpatient programs have tighter control over the supervision of your prescribed regimen. Depending on the program, you may be required to stay in or near the clinic for anywhere from ten days to several weeks. During this time the inpatient team focuses intently on your physical and mental adjustment to your new pain-management attitudes and strategies. Round-the-clock attention and accommodations are costly, however, and so many people prefer outpatient clinics.

The pain-control programs offered through outpatient clinics are similar in content to inpatient ones, except you do not receive such intensive and concentrated attention. You are given scheduled appointments over a period of several weeks or even years depending on your needs. This approach is less demanding and disruptive of your daily life, but it requires more personal commitment from you to go home and practice what you've learned without anyone looking over your shoulder.

In the end, inpatient or outpatient, the goal of a pain clinic is to prepare you to manage your pain on your own without health-care providers recording your every move.

MANAGEMENT GOALS

Because chronic pain is a complex ailment, clinics generally offer a multidisciplinary approach for evaluating and treating this pain. The primary focus of treatment typically is on rehabilitation rather than simply on eradication of symptoms. Restoration of function is especially important for medically stable patients with chronic benign pain (the largest group of chronic pain patients). The functional impairment and disruption of lifestyle that are associated with chronic pain frequently have a larger impact on quality of life than the experience of pain itself. Additionally, the chronic nature of the disorder must be recognized, and you must make a conceptual shift away from a focus on the treatment of acute disease to the management of chronic symptoms. A management approach directly confronts unrealistic expectations (maybe your pain can never be "cured"), reinforces the goal of optimal quality of life given the parameters of chronic disease, and provides a model by which patients may understand their pain and guide their efforts at pain relief and restoration of function. Ultimately, this approach encourages self-management of chronic pain and associated symptoms, with appropriate education and assistance from doctors, therapists, and clinicians.

STAFF MEMBERS

On staff at pain clinics generally are a number of specialists who deal the with the bones, the nerves, and the mind. These specialists often include algologists (pain specialists), anesthesiologists, neurologists, physical and occupational therapists, psychiatrists, and psychologists. Clinics also may have an acupuncturist, osteopath, chiropractor, nutritionist, or any other specialist who may be helpful in diagnosing and treating pain. This team approach reduces the chances that factors such as a rare disease, a personality disorder, or patient/physician incompatibility will interfere with proper treatment.

Algologists often supervise the clinic and treatment plans of each patient. The algologist or attending physician will meet with you to take your medical history, conduct the initial physical exam, talk about your previous pain-control regimens, and finally determine a multidisciplinary course of treatment.

Anesthesiologists are available if patients need short-term pain control. A person suffering from rheumatoid arthritis, for example, may need an injection of a nerve block medication for temporary relief while he or she begins the prescribed exercise plan that eventually will offer drug-free mobility.

Neurologists are on staff to help diagnose and treat pain caused by pressure on a nerve center or pain affecting the nervous system. Occasionally neurosurgeons are called in to operate on the brain or spinal cord.

Physical and occupational therapists are of great help to patients needing training in appropriate posture and body mechanics. These professionals will teach you how to perform appropriate exercises, help you establish a program and routine, and monitor your use of special equipment when necessary. They also can teach you to use other pain-relief methods such as heat and cold treatments and transcutaneous electrical nerve stimulation (TENS).

Psychiatrists and psychologists are integral team members. They use cognitive and behavioral therapies to wean patients from bad habits that perpetuate pain. They teach stress management and relaxation exercises such as meditation, guided visual imagry, autogenic training, and hypnosis, and monitor results with biofeedback. They offer family and marital counseling. They often supervise drug withdrawal.

This is just a sampling of the staff members in a pain clinic. Different combinations of different specialists and technicians may be available at the various pain clinics around the country. Whatever the combination, all work to help their patients reach the therapeutic goal of self-controlled pain management.

THE GOOD AND THE BAD
ABOUT PAIN CLINICS

There is good news and bad news to tell about the surging numbers of pain clinics in recent years. The bad news first: Unfortunately, the success rate of these clinics has been receiving negative publicity. But this is not surprising, considering that most pain-treatment programs do not regularly assess whether patients actually engage in the recommended behaviors. Rather, adherence is inferred on the basis of outcome measures. If patients report that they are more active and less depressed, it is assumed that these results are a function of continued performance of the recommended behaviors. The lack of documented behavioral changes severely limits conclusions regarding the effective ingredients within the treatment programs.

Another reason pain clinics may, indeed, have poor success rates has more to do with the patients than with the effectiveness of the program. Several studies illustrate that considering the typical pain patient, expectations for success may be too high. Many pain-treatment programs are conducted in tightly structured hospital environments and are of relatively brief duration (three to eight weeks). Perhaps we cannot realistically expect long-term changes from short-term treatment in controlled environments. This is especially true when we consider that many chronic pain patients have long-standing histories of inactivity, deconditioning, feelings of helplessness and hopelessness, and a lifetime history of dependence on the health-care system.

Now the good news: The existence of these clinics gives chronic pain sufferers an opportunity to validate their complaint of pain and to do something about it personally. When you walk through the doors of a pain clinic, there are people there who will agree with you: "Yes, chronic pain is a serious medical, emotional, social, and family problem requiring a focused team of specialists." A pain clinic is a place you can go without feeling that you are imposing on a busy doctor's time; you'll feel "Yes, chronic pain sufferers have legitimate complaints; they are not hypocondriacs, lazy, or willing drug abusers." Also, pain clinics offer a multidisciplined noninvasive approach to pain management; you can go there without worrying that you're in for more invasive testing, drugs, or surgery. Instead, you'll learn new and effective techniques for reducing the frequency and intensity of your pain. You'll learn how to treat your pain without habit-forming narcotic analgesic and sedative drugs. And you'll establish a positive outlook that will enable you to take what you learn in the clinic out into your world where you can get on with a life that includes chronic pain as one of its many facets—not its main focus. And finally, and in the long run very important, pain clinics are much more cost effective than conventional medical approaches.

Pain clinics are now relatively readily available throughout the United States. To find a clinic, you can ask your doctor for a referral. Or you can call your nearest university hospital and ask to be directed to a pain clinic in your area.

FINDING A GOOD CLINIC

When you find a pain clinic, you should interview the director before you sign up for treatment. Take a tour of the facility and ask lots of questions. Here are some areas you should consider.

• A good clinic will be staffed by a multidisciplinary team as outlined earlier in this chapter; find out exactly who will be part of your management team.

• Question how chronic pain patients are evaluated and chosen for clinic treatment: Will your medical history be reviewed, and will you receive a comprehensive physical and psychological evaluation before you begin any therapy?

• Some noninvasive treatments are quite high tech; ask if the clinic has biofeedback machines, physical therapy equipment, and exercise apparatus.

• There should be one particular team member you can talk to on a regular basis. Find out how often you will meet with this person to discuss your progress. Ask how often your treatment plan will be reviewed and changed as needed.

• Your family should be considered a part of your treatment team. Ask if they will be included in your counseling.

• There is no *one* remedy that will manage the pain of chronic ailments and diseases. Find out exactly what therapies are offered at the clinic. Compare those therapies to the ones detailed in Chapter 3. The clinic should offer a wide range of these natural therapies.

The Commission on Accreditation of Rehabilitation Facilities (CARF) supervises the accreditation of chronic pain clinics across the country. Although there are many legitimate pain clinics not accredited by CARF, you can get a free list of the programs they have approved by writing:

The CARF Report
2500 North Pantano Road
Tuscon, AZ 85715

A pain clinic is a place to go for help and direction as you implement the natural therapies outlined in this book. But remember: Your conscientious adherence to your prescribed treatment regimen is absolutely vital to your evaluation of the clinic's success or failure. No pain clinic, no doctor, no drug, not anything or anyone can make your chronic pain manageable. Only you can do that. The information in this book is offered as tools to assist you, as encouragement to support you, and as information to guide you. But in the end, it's your commitment to taking control of your own life and the management of your pain that will determine how well natural medicine can improve the quality of your life.

Good luck. We know you can do it.

Glossary

acetaminophen: A chemical that can reduce pain and fever but does not have the anti-inflammatory properties of aspirin.

acute pain: Pain that usually lasts less than six months; pain subsides as healing takes place.

analgesic: Any compound that relieves pain without producing anesthesia or loss of consciousness.

arthritis: A group of diseases affecting joints or their component tissues.

brachial neuralgia: Peripheral nerve damage caused by strained physical exercise, exposure to severe cold, or accumulation of fatigue after heavy labor.

chronic pain: A term usually used to refer to any pain that lasts six months or longer.

cordotomy: A surgical procedure in which the neurosurgeon inserts an electric needle into the spinal cord and congeals the nerve tract that carries fibers from the affected area through the spine to the brain.

degenerative arthritis: A disease of the aging process that involves degeneration of cartilage and joints.

degenerative disk disease: A condition affecting the back caused by the aging process and resulting in pain and disability.

dorsal column stimulation: A technique for the relief of chronic pain, based on the gate control theory of pain.

dorsal rhizotomy: A neurosurgical procedure in which the surgeon cuts the roots of the nerves connecting the spinal cord with a specific part of the anatomy.

drug tolerance: After repeated doses, a given dosage of a narcotic begins to lose its effectiveness.

electrode implants: Electrodes surgically placed just behind the spinal cord to cause electrically stimulated interference with the passage of substance P through the gate mechanism.

electrostimulation: An attempt to make the nerves resistant to pain in which a neurosurgeon inserts an electric needle into the spinal cord and stimulates the nerve fibers.

endorphin: A naturally produced chemical that has a morphinelike action.

gate theory: An attempt to explain the mechanism by which an overloaded pathway to the brain will selectively eliminate the painful transmission.

herniated disk: A back problem caused by rupture of the spinal disk core through its outer fiber covering.

hysterical pain: Pain that is a symptom of or results from unconscious emotional conflicts that have their origins in the past.

inflammatory arthritis: A subgroup of arthritis characterized by inflammation of joint fluid and the surrounding tissue, including connective tissue diseases, rheumatoid arthritis, crystal deposition diseases, infectious arthritis, and spondyloarthropathies.

intercostal neuralgia: A condition causing pain along the nerve pathways in the chest region.

intractable pain: Pain that persists despite treatment.

lumbar neuralgia: A condition causing pain along the nerve pathways in the lower back.

metastatic disease: A disease that spreads from an afflicted point to other parts of the body.

migraine headache: A vascular headache of such intensity that it can be incapacitating.

musculoskeletal pain syndrome: A variety of symptoms, including pain, caused by abnormal pressure of muscles and bones on adjacent nerves.

myofascial pain dysfunction: Pain or discomfort caused by inflammation of the tissue that surrounds many muscles in the head, neck, and jaw area.

narcotic: A drug derived from opium or opiumlike compounds that can affect mood, behavior, and the perception of pain, and has a potential for dependence and tolerance.

nerve block: A method of arresting the passage of pain signals usually by injecting a chemical into the nerve.

neuralgia: Nerve pain that feels like severe throbbing or stabbing along the nerve pathway.

nonarticular rheumatism: A catch-all term for various types of arthritis including tendonitis, bursitis, tenosynovitis, fibrositis, and psychogenic rheumatism.

noninvasive pain-relief methods: Techniques that can be used to relieve pain without physically invading or penetrating the body.

NSAID: An acronym for a nonsteroidal anti-inflammatory drug, such as aspirin.

occipital neuralgia: A condition causing pain in the back of the head along the nerve path from the hairline on the neck up to the area behind the ears.

opiate: Any chemical derived from opium that produces pain relief.

organic pain: Pain sensations that result from a physical source.

over-the-counter drugs: Medications available to consumers without prescriptions from medical doctors.

pain behavior: Anything that a person does or says that communicates that pain is being experienced.

pain clinic: A pain-treatment center that involves the input of a multidisciplinary team that treats the physical causes of pain as well as its psychological components.

postherpetic neuralgia: Any irritation or inflammation of a nerve that is the result of an infection caused by the herpes virus.

psychogenic pain: A localized sensation of pain that originates in the mind: that is, no physical findings exist to account for the cause of the pain.

reflex sympathetic dystrophy: A disorder of the sympathetic nervous system.

rheumatoid arthritis: A chronic inflammatory disease that affects mainly the connective tissue of the joints.

spondylolisthesis: A condition caused by a defect in the spinal arch that results in the sliding forward of one vertebra onto the one below it.

substance P: A neurotransmitter that carries pain signals to the brain.

temporomandibular joint: A joint located between the bones of the skull and the lower jaw. Damage to the joint, either by excessive grinding of the teeth or by injury to the muscle attaching the jaw to the skull, can create a painful syndrome called temporomandibular joint syndrome (TMJ).

transcutaneous electrical nerve stimulation (TENS): Stimulation of nerves through electrodes placed over the skin and activated by a battery-operated device to provide tingling or vibrating sensations in the area of pain.

trigeminal neuralgia (tic douloureux):   An irritation of one of the nerves in the face.

trigger point: Hypersensitive regions that may occur in muscles, connective tissue, ligaments, and joint capsules.

Natural Medicine Resources

American Association of Acupuncture and Oriental Medicine
4101 Lake Boone Trail, Suite 201
Raleigh, NC 27607-6528
(919) 965-7546

American Association of Naturopathic Physicians
P.O. Box 2579
Kirkland, WA 98083-2579
(206) 827-6035

American Association of Orthomolecular Medicine
900 North Federal Highway, Suite 330
Boca Raton, FL 33432
(407) 276-6167

American Chiropractic Association
17021 Clarendon Boulevard
Arlington, VA 22209
(703) 276-8800

American Foundation for Alternative Health Care, Research and Development
25 Landfield Avenue
Monticello, NY 12701
(914) 794-8181

American Herb Association
P.O. Box 535
Rescue, CA 95672

American Holistic Medical Association
2727 Fairview Avenue East, Suite B
Seattle, WA 98102
(206) 322-6842

American Massage Therapy Association
National Information Office
1130 West North Shore Avenue
Chicago, IL 60626
(312) 761-2682

Biofeedback Certification Institute of America
10200 West 44th Avenue, #304
Wheat Ridge, CO 80033
(303) 420-2902

Center for Medical Consumers
237 Thompson Street
New York, NY 10012
(212) 674-7105

Human Nutrition Center
6303 Ivy Lane
Greenbelt, MD 20770
(301) 344-2340

**International Academy of Nutrition and Preventive
    Medicine**
P.O. Box 5832
Lincoln, NE 68505
(402) 467-2716

International Institute of Reflexology
P.O. Box 12462

St. Petersburg, FL 33733
(813) 343-4811

International Pain Foundation
909 NE 43rd Street, Suite 306
Seattle, WA 98105
(206) 547-2157

Integral Yoga Institute
227 West 13th Street
New York, NY 10011
(212) 929-0586

**National Accreditation Commission for Schools and
    Colleges of Acupuncture and Oriental Medicine**
8403 Colesville Road, Suite 370
Silver Spring, MD 20919
(301) 608-9680

National Center for Homeopathy
801 North Fairfax, Suite 306
Alexandria, VA 22314
(703) 548-7790

**National Commission for the Certification of
    Acupuncturists**
1424 16 Street NW, Suite 501
Washington, DC 20036
(202) 232-1404

National Headache Foundation
5252 North Western Avenue
Chicago, IL 60625
(800) 843-2256

Herb Sources

Annandale Apothecary
7023 Little River Turnpike
Annandale, VA 22003

Boerick and Tafel, Inc.
1011 Arch Street
Philadelphia, PA 19107
or
2381 Circadian Way
Santa Rosa, CA 95407

Boiron-Borneman, Inc.
6 Campus Blvd.
Bldg. A
Newtown Square, PA 19073

Ehrhart and Karl
17 North Wabash Avenue
Chicago, IL 60602

Herbarium
264 Exchange Street
Chicopee, MA

Horton and Converse
621 West Pico Blvd.
Los Angeles, CA 90015

Humphreys Pharmacal Company
63 Meadow Road
Rutherford, NJ 07070

Keihl Pharmacy, Inc.
109 Third Avenue
New York, NY 10003

Luyties Pharmacal Company
4200 Laclede Avenue
St. Louis, MO 63108

Mylans Homeopathic Pharmacy
222 O'Farrell Street
San Francisco, CA 94102

Running Fox Farm (flower essences)
74 Thrashing Hill Road
Worthington, MA 01098
(413) 238-4291

Santa Monica Drug
1513 Fourth Street
Santa Monica, CA 90401

Standard Homeopathic Company
204–210 West 131 Street
Los Angeles, CA 90061

Washington Homeopathic Pharmacy
4914 Delray Avenue
Bethesda, MD 20814

Weleda, Inc.
841 South Main Street
Spring Valley, NY 10977

Acupressure Points

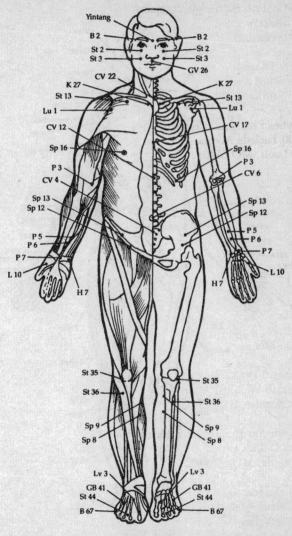

Front View

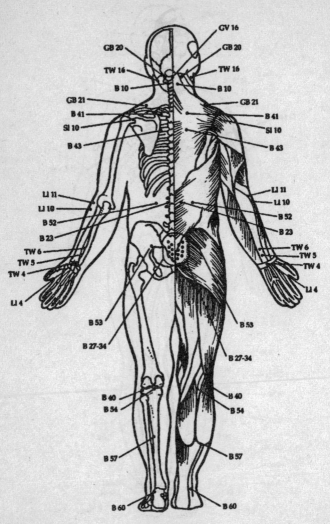

Back View

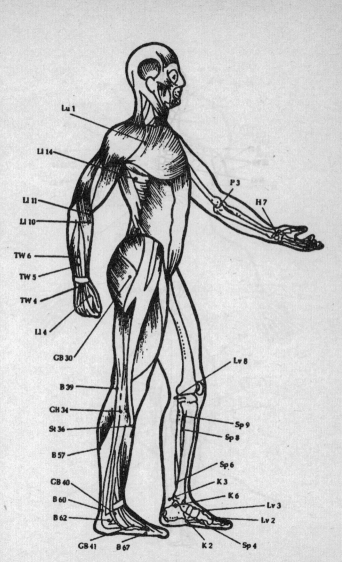

Side View

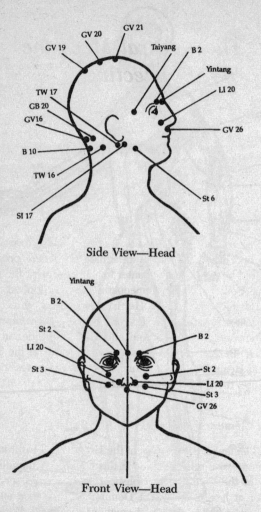

Side View—Head

Front View—Head

The Natural Medicine Collective:

BIOGRAPHIES

Dr. William Bergman (*Homeopathy*)

William Bergman holds an M.D. degree from Columbia University and has completed postgraduate physicians' programs sponsored by the National Center for Homeopathy, the International Foundation for Homeopathy, and the United States Homeopathic Association. He is the medical director of Hahnemann Health Associates, one of the most comprehensive homeopathic medical and educational facilities in New York. Dr. Bergman also serves as the president of the World Medical Health Foundation, Inc., an organization researching the cause, treatment, and prevention of disease.

Brian Clement (*Nutrition*)

Brian Clement is the director of the Hippocrates Institute, the first progressive health center in this country. A founding director of the Coalition of Holistic Health, he has served as director at health centers in Denmark and Greece and has consulted at holistic clinics throughout the world. With over twenty years of international leadership experience in the field of alternative health care, he has appeared on numerous radio and television shows and has conducted hundreds of workshops and seminars on natural medicine.

Dr. Brian Fradet *(Chiropractic, Panel Coordinator)*

Brian Fradet holds a doctorate of chiropractic from the prestigious New York Chiropractic College and has completed postgraduate research in neurology at the New York University Medical Center. He is a longstanding member of the American Chiropractic Association, the Foundation for Chiropractic Education and Research, the Parker Chiropractic Research Foundation, the New York State Chiropractic Association, and the Chiropractic Federated Society of New York. He is the founder of the Fradet Pain Clinic in New York.

Elaine Retholtz, L.Ac. *(Acupuncture)*

Elaine Retholtz is a licensed acupuncturist and a diplomate of the National Commission for the Certification of Acupuncturists. She is a graduate of the Tri-State Institute of Traditional Chinese Acupuncture. She holds a master's degree in nutritional sciences from the University of Wisconsin-Madison. She maintains a private practice in New York specializing in acupuncture. She is the supervising acupuncturist for Crossroads: An Alternative for Women Offenders—A Project of the Center for Community Alternatives (formerly National Center on Institutions and Alternatives/Northeast).

Dr. James Lawrence Thomas *(Psychology)*

James Lawrence Thomas is a licensed psychologist and neuropsychologist with postdoctoral certificates in cognitive, relationship, group, and brief therapy. He is on the faculty of the New York University Medical Center and has served as the consulting neuropsychologist to Mt. Sinai Medical Center's Department of Neurology. He holds degrees from Yale, the

University of California, Berkeley, and City University of New York. Dr. Thomas maintains a private practice in New York.

Dr. Maurice H. Werness, Jr. *(Naturopathy)*

Maurice H. Werness, Jr. received a doctoral degree from the Bastyr College of Naturopathic Medicine. He is the medical director of HEALINGHEART HEALTHCARE, one of the West Coast's most prominent facilities for holistic care. He is also the director of development at the Institute for Naturopathic Medicine. A former tennis professional, Dr. Werness is the founder and director of True Tennis, an organization that teaches tennis and health education to physically and emotionally challenged people.

Theresa DiGeronimo, M.Ed., is an adjunct professor of English at the William Paterson College of New Jersey. She has collaborated on numerous health-care books, including the award-winning *AIDS: Trading Fears for Facts*. She lives in New Jersey with her husband and three children.

Index